MEDICINE IN THE ENGLISH MIDDLE AGES

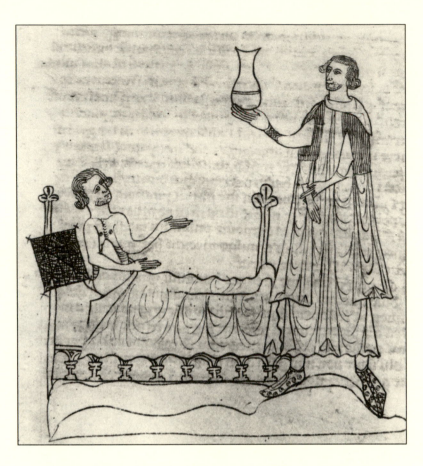

Uroscopy. Thirteenth-century English manuscript. Cambridge, King's College, MS 21, p. 149. (Courtesy of the Provost and Fellows of King's College, Cambridge.)

MEDICINE
IN THE ENGLISH
MIDDLE AGES

Faye Getz

PRINCETON UNIVERSITY PRESS   PRINCETON, NEW JERSEY

Copyright ©1998 by Princeton University Press
Published by Princeton University Press, 41 William Street,
Princeton, New Jersey 08540
In the United Kingdom: Princeton University Press,
Chichester, West Sussex
All Rights Reserved

Library of Congress Cataloging-in-Publication Data

Getz, Faye Marie, 1952–
Medicine in the English Middle Ages / Faye Getz.
p.   cm.
Includes bibliographical references and index.
ISBN 0-691-08522-6 (cl : alk. paper)
1. Medicine, Medieval—England—History. 2. Medicine—
England—History. I. Title.
R487.G47   1998
160′.942′0902—dc21   98-3534

This book has been composed in New Baskerville

Princeton University Press books are printed
on acid-free paper and meet the guidelines
for permanence and durability of the Committee
on Production Guidelines for Book Longevity
of the Council on Library Resources

http://pup.princeton.edu

Printed in the United States of America

1   3   5   7   9   10   8   6   4   2

For Hal

When a man has sinned against his Maker
Let him put himself in the doctor's hands.

(*Ecclesiasticus 38:15*)

Contents

THE TRIUMPH of modern scientific medicine in contemporary Western culture has been so complete we often forget that, before science, the person wishing to preserve or regain good health was presented with many alternatives, none of which was entirely satisfactory from a modern point of view. The ways of our early ancestors may seem foolish to us: herbalism, philosophical advice, magic, or so-called folk remedies—all of which seem to be based on luck, superstition, or error. But no person living in a prescientific culture could be expected to count scientific medicine among his or her many healing choices. If we find the medieval medical patron's obsession with uroscopy or astrology, for instance, to be bizarre or amusing, and wonder why anyone took such methods seriously, then we must also remember that these methods were, like the medical patron, firmly rooted in a particular time and place. In this context, astrological medicine is best understood not as irrational and erroneous but rather as a complex system of explanations, many of which could be justified empirically or historically, based on a particular society's beliefs about the functioning of the natural world.

Claude Lévi-Strauss, in his *Structural Anthropology*, studied the role of the shaman, or traditional healer, among the Kwakiutl Indians of the Vancouver region.[1] He postulated what he called the "shamanistic complex" to explain the remarkable success of the shaman among his or her people. This complex consisted of the healer, the afflicted, and what he called the "social consensus." The belief of the healer's audience (which included the afflicted) in the success of the healing practice was more important than any other factor in determining the secure place of a particular shaman in his or her culture. Whether a particular practice "really" worked, then, was much less important than the audience's belief that it had. A healer, Lévi-Strauss concluded, "did not become a great shaman because he cured his patients; he cured his patients because he had become a great shaman."[2]

The work of Lévi-Strauss and others confronts one of the most troubling aspects of the history of medicine in prescientific culture: why did people adhere to practices that modern science finds nonsensical? The anthropologist answers that this happened because of the social consensus that such practices were effective. And the social consensus of any culture must derive from the complexities of the culture itself.

In any culture, the reputation of the healer is vital for these practices to flourish. Medicine, like poetry, required an audience to grow. Medical learning in medieval England from about 750 to about 1450 is the focus of

this book, and the central argument concerns how this learning, understood as the medicine that was written down in texts, gained an audience
among English people. The struggles of learned physicians to establish a
reputation for themselves and for their medicine are an important part of
this argument, as are the public character of health and disease, and the
struggle of the medical practitioner to develop an audience for medical
learning, especially among the elite of later medieval English culture. Evidence from medical texts, university and church records, legal documents,
and literary sources have proven rich resources for this study. But as valu-
able as these primary sources have been, the work of other historians and
social scientists has been even more useful. The world of medieval English
medical culture is complex, too complex for one historian to grasp. History
is a collective enterprise, and the debt any of us owes to the labors of others
cannot be ignored. The achievements of past scholars make me humble,
and my work is built on theirs.

Cooksville, Wisconsin

Acknowledgments

RESEARCH for this publication was funded in part by NIH Grant LM005144 from the National Library of Medicine. It was also funded with the assistance of a grant for college teachers and independent scholars from the National Endowment for the Humanities. I am deeply grateful to both agencies for their faith and support.

Edward Tenner solicited the book manuscript and Lauren Osborne made invaluable suggestions along the way. Brigitta van Rheinberg guided the book to completion with uncommon skill and total professionalism. I would also like to thank Princeton's production staff, especially Kim Mrazek Hastings, who copy edited the text superbly. Katharine Park and an anonymous reader made suggestions for improvement that were offered with both tact and wisdom. Much that is good in this book can be attributed to their time and learning. Nothing that is bad can be blamed on anyone but me.

I would also like to thank the libraries of the Wellcome Institute for the History of Medicine in London, the Institute of Historical Research, the Warburg Institute, and the Public Record Office; the British Library, the Middleton and Memorial Libraries of the University of Wisconsin-Madison, the Bodleian Library, and the library of Leiden University, The Netherlands.

Part of chapter 3 appeared in an earlier version in *Roger Bacon and the Sciences*, edited by Jeremiah Hackett (Leiden: E. J. Brill, 1997). Part of chapter 4 appeared in an earlier version in *The History of Medical Education in Britain*, edited by Vivian Nutton and Roy Porter (Amsterdam: Rodopi, 1995). Both are reproduced by permission.

Peter Murray Jones selected the illustration for this book. It would not have been possible without his unfailing friendship and professional support.

The generosity offered by members of the academic community made it possible for me to continue my work even without a job. So many have shown me collegiality throughout the years that they cannot all be named. I am especially grateful to Keith Benson, Mario Biagioli, James Bono, Allan Brandt, Joan Cadden, the late William Coleman, William Courtenay, Ralph Drayton, William Eamon, Mordechai Feingold, Eric Freeman, A. Rupert Hall, Marie Boas Hall, Caroline Hannaway, Stanley Jackson, Stuart Jenks, David Lindberg, Michael MacDonald, Michael R. McVaugh, Robert Martensen, John Neu, Nicholas Orme, Margaret Pelling, Roy Porter, Shirley Roe, Walton O. Schalick, Jane Schulenburg, Nancy Siraisi, the late Charles

Talbot, Godelieve Van Heteren, Linda Ehrsam Voigts, John Harley Warner, and Charles Webster.

I also would like to thank my friends, who never failed to take me seriously as a scholar, whether I deserved it or not: Dorothy Africa, the Beukers family, Martha Carlin, Cathy Cornish, the Kerkhoff family, David Harris Sacks, and Eleanor Sacks. I regret that my friend Gemmie Beukers, of Leiderdorp, The Netherlands, did not live to see the completion of one more scholar's work that her hospitality made easier. Her untimely death makes the world a less civilized place, and she is mourned by all who knew her.

Finally, I am happy to thank my husband, Harold Cook. His high scholarly ideals and devotion to workplace equality have served as an example for his many students, among whom I count myself. All that is good in this book is dedicated to him.

MEDICINE IN THE ENGLISH MIDDLE AGES

CHAPTER I

The Variety of Medical Practitioners
in Medieval England

IN THE SUMMER of 1205, Hubert Walter, archbishop of Canterbury, suddenly fell ill with a deadly fever and carbuncle (*anthrax*) while traveling to Boxley in Kent. So severe was his illness that he was forced to divert to a nearby manor of his, Teynham. The carbuncle erupted around his waist, at the third-from-last vertebra of his back, with the inflammation extending around so as to threaten his private parts.

The archbishop, a remarkable lawyer who helped develop Henry II's legal and financial system, had accompanied Henry's son Richard the Lion-Hearted on a crusade to Palestine. In his illness, Hubert was attended by Master Gilbert Eagle (Gillbertus del Egle, also called Gilbertus Anglicus), a medical authority whose career was in its own way no less remarkable. Gilbert, from a prominent Essex family, may have visited the Holy Land himself. He attended Richard's brother John, was summoned to Rome in 1214 for continuing to perform priestly duties while England was under the Interdict of Innocent III, and was the author of a massive medical and surgical text, the *Compendium medicine* (Compendium of medicine), one of the first works to take advantage of new Latin translations of Arabic medical and philosophical texts.

Gilbert, worried that his patron's fever would rise, advised him to confess his sins. On doing so, the fire of the archbishop's remorse and charity rose up and caused the moisture in his brain to dissolve, bringing forth from him a torrent of tears and great relief. After this, he was able to eat and drink a bit. Gilbert then advised him to make out his will, which he did in good order. At dawn the next day, Gilbert secretly observed the ill man and advised Hubert to receive last rites. Another physician, Henry le Afaitie, disagreed and advised him to wait. The poisonous matter that was causing the fever then went to the archbishop's brain and he became delirious. He had to be brought back to himself with "physical remedies" (*remedia physicalia*) and shortly thereafter followed Gilbert's advice.

After last rites, Hubert was much relieved, and joined others in praying and rejoicing. He was also able to conclude some last matters of business before fever returned and weariness overcame him. He could not be roused either by friends or by medicines. There was no medicine for this kind of weariness (*languor*) but death alone, for disease sapped his body of vitality, and the furnace of fevers compelled his soul to leave the seat of the body at last.[1]

The chronicler of this dramatic episode, Ralph of Coggeshall, was anxious for his readers to understand that the archbishop of Canterbury had not died intestate, as some had asserted. Far from it; Hubert's death was a tidy one, with things done in the correct order at the correct time. Ralph described each event on the day and canonical hour it unfolded ("at prime," "after vespers," etc.), and the only disruption in the archbishop's procession to his death came from a medical practitioner who put "physical remedies" ahead of spiritual ones. The author of Hubert's orderly passing was the most famous physician of his time. But Gilbert administered not a single drug, nor was he said to have viewed the dying man's urine or to have taken his pulse. Instead, the great doctor exercised his peerless judgment, knowing his master so intimately that he could tell by a glance that death was at hand. Confession, not potions, brought the archbishop relief, and the oil of the last rites enabled Hubert to take care of worldly matters before the inevitable stilled the hand of the renowned cleric and man of affairs forever. Gilbert was presented as the hero of this episode, not because he saved the archbishop, but because he used his learned judgment to recognize that death was unavoidable, and that the life of a great man must be shepherded to its end with ritual and dignity.

Gilbert's doubtless heroism reminds one more of King Arthur or Theseus than it does of Pasteur or Salk. Gilbert in this telling anecdote was presented as the master of time and the bringer of order, not the deliverer of mere physical remedies. Like all learned physicians of his day, Gilbert was an astrologer, which allowed him not to predict the future but to recognize the stages of progress according to God's will and as a consequence of humanity's actions. What is more, as an Aristotelian philosopher, Gilbert was not distracted by the "accidents," or side effects, of the process of dying. Instead, he concentrated his learned judgment on the important issue before him—a decorous exit from the physical world for the archbishop's immortal soul.

We do not now think of the duties of the medical professions in this way. The universals of disease, suffering, and death unite us with the distant past, but the "otherness" exposed by stories like that of Gilbert and the archbishop must inevitably draw us away from facile comparisons. The welfare of the soul lies outside the modern medical practitioner's purview: the priest, physician, friend, and adviser are nowadays not the same person. In an age before scientific medicine, a medical practitioner was almost never simply a practitioner. Instead, he or she could perform a number of different functions, not all of which we associate with medical practice. A survey of these medical practitioners therefore opens up issues of social status, gender, literacy, income, institutional affiliation, and relationship to sources of patronage. And yet, much as such an approach may promise, medieval English healers defy any easy attempts at classification or characterization. Were men like Gilbert primarily physicians, or were they rather philosophers, priests, or teachers? And what about the less elite medical practitioners? What was the range of their activities?

The most distinctive feature of medieval English medicine is indeed the variety of people who practiced it. Unlike other medieval professions that survive today—the ministry, legal and notarial arts, and teaching—medieval medical practice embraced men and women, serfs and free people, Christians and non-Christians, academics and tradespeople, the wealthy and the poor, the educated and those ignorant of formal learning. Such a wide diversity among healers suggests that the term "profession" cannot be applied to medieval English medical practice in any meaningful way.

Terms like "profession" gain their meaning from the way scholars use them. Judged by this standard, medieval England lacked a medical profession. One major work on the professions in medieval England omits medicine entirely.[2] Histories of the professions in the early modern period (from about 1500 to 1700) have been more forthcoming, drawing attention away from the traditional emphasis on a few university-educated doctors and embracing a variety of tradespeople.[3] Some have suggested that the term "medical profession" in the sixteenth and seventeenth centuries is deceptive, since it ignores the diversity of types of practitioners, the lack of social consensus about standards of conduct, and the domination of medical practice by people who acted only part-time.[4] Harold Cook has argued that during the sixteenth and seventeenth centuries a scholastically educated medical elite exerted legal authority over medical practice in a way it never had in medieval England. Even so, the powerful London College of Physicians was not a professional monopoly, but rather one of many competitors in England's "medical marketplace," albeit the most powerful one, whose fortunes rose and fell according not to superior healing abilities but to the growth in the monarchy's public power.[5]

What early modernists have suggested for their period by and large holds true for medieval England as well. No single group of practitioners distinguished itself by force of numbers, by healing skill, or by civic sanction as a dominant medical profession.[6] Although the structure of trade guilds and university education helped set a certain standard of conduct in a commercial and legal sphere for a few practicers, the vast majority of medics operated independently, and, from the educated elite to the tradesperson, often part-time. This allowed for diversity of every sort, which changed little throughout the medieval period and beyond.[7]

Most people involved in medical learning or practice, then, fell under no particular heading. They might have involved themselves in medicine only on occasion, written about it as a part of general knowledge, or healed as a religious duty. Others were independent tradespeople: nurses, midwives, toothdrawers, or country practitioners, whose training and methods varied enormously. Most medicine must have been practiced by the family or by neighbors, whose lives and methods remain hidden.[8]

The historical sources for the lives of all medical people in medieval England are of course found in written documents and are as a consequence biased toward the famous or the notorious. Learned physicians and surgeons sometimes composed texts containing biographical details about themselves, their friends, and their rivals. The university-educated man left his mark in institutional documents, whereas people in organized trade were enrolled in guild registers or called upon by municipal officials for expert opinion. We also have the records of payments given to doctors who attended clerics and royal or noble persons. The ordinary practitioner, however, is most often known indirectly through legal documents, either as a party in the transfer of property or as a litigant. Knowledge about people involved in medicine is therefore very incomplete, especially with regard to women, who could enter into the records of the law, university, and church only rarely, and yet by their patronage showed themselves to be both knowledgeable about and interested in medicine.[9]

One way of thinking about the various types of medical practitioners is to divide them into tradespeople or ordinary practitioners and clerical or elite practitioners. These divisions should be thought of not as rigid categories but rather as polarities: clerical practitioners often had the characteristics of tradespeople, and tradespeople at times adopted some trappings of clerical practitioners, especially with regard to the ownership or production of surgical texts.

Medical tradespeople practiced medicine in the same way people did any other trade. They sold care and drugs sometimes as a member of a guild or with the license of a municipal authority. Sometimes they worked for a monastery, or in a royal or noble household. Some solicited clients on the street or worked from a shop. The great majority were free men or women, but there are occasional records of serfs practicing medicine. The tradesperson/medical practitioner could receive payment for services in cash, either in the form of an annuity or for services rendered. Many were given gifts, especially of clothing and food. The practice of medicine in return for payment is found on all social levels throughout the medieval period.[10]

The clerical practitioner dealt not in payment for services but in healing as a part of clerical duty. Even the religious required material support, however, and the clerical practitioner derived income not directly from clients but from the church. Powerful patrons were able to gain multiple ecclesiastical incomes for their favorites, and the clerical practitioner was no exception: many royal doctors were notable pluralists, holding multiple incomes, sometimes to the outrage of the less generously endowed. Courtly medical practitioners gained similar preferments from royal and noble prerogatives. But in theory, at least, the clerical practitioner lived in imitation of Christ, and dispensed the healing that could come only from God in the same way he dispensed the sacraments—as a part of charitable duty.[11]

ORDINARY PRACTITIONERS ALONE AND IN FAMILY-LIKE GROUPS

The ordinary practitioner or tradesperson should no doubt be the principal focus of any study of the variety of medical practitioners in medieval England, and yet it is this person about whom the least is known. References to the independent medical tradesperson, both urban and rural, occur frequently throughout the medieval period but are almost always incidental to nonmedical matters. Charles Talbot and Eugene Hammond, in their biographical register of medieval English practitioners, have noticed in taxation records from the late thirteenth century for the city of Worcester that among nearly ten thousand names only three are called physicians.[12] This suggests that medical care, if given by medical practitioners at all, was provided by people recognizable as such only occasionally.

For example, Richard Knyght, known because of the complex trail of litigation he left in London courts during the middle of the fifteenth century—some of it in conjunction with his brother John, a tailor—was known variously as *ffecissian* (physician), ironmonger, surgeon, and *dogleche* (dog doctor).[13] He seems to have practiced his various vocations on his own, not as part of any group.

Some seem to have practiced medicine independently by soliciting patients on the street. The record of the court of John of Preston, sheriff of London, states that one John of Cornhill approached Alice of Stocking on Fleet Street, London, in June 1320. Claiming to be a surgeon ("ad eam accessit usurpando sibi officium surgici"), he offered to cure her of a malady of the feet. As a result of his treatment, she claimed, she was unable to put her feet to the ground. While she was bedridden, John entered her dwelling and stole bedclothes and clothing. Alice was awarded damages of more than £30.[14]

Very little work has been done on medical care in agrarian communities, but legal documents do give occasional hints of medical practitioners performing healing at least part-time. For example, in a charter establishing a Cistercian abbey at Revesby, Lincolnshire, in 1143, one of the tenants displaced from the new abbey's lands was called William, *medicus.* He seems to have been a serf.[15]

Other independent practitioners seem to have engaged in a variety of trades. In 1327 the Italian *fiscisien* Francisco de Massa Sancti Petri, who practiced in London, was a party in a petition to the king revealing his involvement in the wool trade.[16] In 1348 the London surgeon Henry de Rochester left his brewery on Barbican Street to his wife Johanna.[17] Another brewer-physician was a certain William who in 1325 was fined 2s. 8d. (2 shillings and 8 pence) for "brewing and selling" without a license in Lancashire.[18]

Essex country doctor John Crophill made his principal living not from medical practice but from his duties as bailiff (acting principally as a rent collector) for a Benedictine nunnery in the mid-fifteenth century. He also was appointed ale taster for the local lord of the manor, both of which duties left him ample time for a popular medical practice.[19] The gift to Crophill of some ale tankards from a local friar occasioned a drinking party, at which the doctor made dedication speeches in verse to the women present—revealing yet another talent.[20] Elsewhere, Crophill recorded how he brewed ale at his home in Wix.[21]

Surgeons especially seem to have engaged in metalworking as a trade, probably making surgical instruments for themselves and for sale purposes. John Bradmore, the London surgeon, was also called *gemestre*, possibly indicating involvement in the jewelry trade. Bradmore is credited with devising a surgical instrument for the extraction of an arrow from the head of the future Henry V in 1403.[22] Another apparent metalworker was the apothecary (*appotagarius*) John Hexham, who had a shop in London in 1415. He apparently counterfeited coin, for which he was hanged.[23]

The most frequently encountered designations in medieval legal documents are the well-known titles barber (a haircutter who might perform bloodletting or minor surgery on the skin), barber-surgeon (a barber who also performed surgery), leech,[24] *le mire*,[25] *medicus*,[26] *chirurgus* or *sururgicus*,[27] and *physicus*.[28] A rare title is *archiater.*[29] Often one encounters the designation "master" or its Latin translation "magister," which was used both in reference to a master tradesman and to suggest a man who had formal education or was a teacher.[30]

Legal documents use several titles interchangeably throughout the later medieval period, in distinct contrast to more scholarly sources, which employ medical terminology more narrowly. Nicholas Wodehill of London was called surgeon alias leech in a pardon recorded in the patent rolls of 1445, while the same alias was given to another London practitioner called Nicholas about 1272 in an inquisition post mortem.[31] Master Robert, *medicus sive phisicus* (medic or physician), witnessed a London will in 1391.[32] The Winchester practitioner Master Hugh was known as both *medicus* and *physicus* during the late twelfth century and Master John, a Scotsman, was known by both titles in the early thirteenth, as was his fellow Scot, Master Robert, who flourished about 1250.[33] The Westminster Infirmarers' Rolls, which chronicle the various expenses of the monks, seem to use *medicus* and *physicus* indifferently throughout the fourteenth and fifteenth centuries in reference to medical practitioners who came from outside to care for the monks.[34]

The titles barber, barber-surgeon, and surgeon could denote guild associations, and their use reflects the complex history of their respective fellowships. The late-fifteenth-century London practitioner Master Robert Halyday was listed in various documents as barber, barber-surgeon, and surgeon,[35] while Londoners John Child and John Dalton, both of whom flourished around the end of the fourteenth and beginning of the fifteenth centuries, were called both barber and barber-surgeon.[36]

Other titles are encountered among ordinary practitioners as well. Eadricus the phlebotomist (*fleubotomarius*) witnessed a charter in Essex about 1150, whereas a certain John from Essex received a penny a day from the royal exchequer from at least 1156 until 1171, and is called variously *minutor, medicus, dubbedent,* and *adubedent,* indicating designations as a phlebotomist, medic, and toothdrawer.[37] Another toothdrawer was Matthew Flynt of London, who was paid 6d. a day about 1400 by the royal exchequer to treat the poor for free.[38] Marjory Cobbe of Devon, midwife (*obstetrix*), was granted an annual pension of £10 in 1469 for her attendance on Elizabeth, wife of Edward IV,[39] but references to midwives are rare. The 1381 poll tax of the London suburb of Southwark, which stated the occupations of every householder, noted only 1 woman midwife out of 137 female householders listed (by comparison, there was 1 carpenter and 1 mason).[40] Midwives likely practiced their trade independently.

Apothecaries and medical practitioners seem to have substituted for each other on occasion. The apothecary Robert of Montpellier spiced Henry III's wine at the table, but when he was absent, the royal physician Ralph de Neketon did the job.[41] The Italian physician Pancio da Controne was treated in 1329 by several doctors and by the French apothecary Peter of Montpellier.[42]

Both men and women were medical practitioners, but exclusion from the higher levels of the clergy, the university, and independent membership in most medical guilds confined women to the realm of the ordinary independent practitioner. Gender, then, mattered a great deal in medieval English medical practice because it excluded women from the highest levels of elite practice, where the clerical practitioner was the norm. It mattered much less in the middling levels of society, where the tradeswoman might hope to pursue her craft away from interference from the church.

References to women practitioners are uncommon but not absent from legal records.[43] For instance, the court rolls of the manor of Hales in Worcestershire contain several mentions of a certain Margery, called "leech." Margery's existence and vocation are known only from her involvement in several actions before the local manorial court between 1300 and 1306. She was fined three times for damage to the lord's land by allowing her cow to stray and by gathering nuts and firewood without permission. In one case, the fine amounted to 4d. In 1302, however, she herself, with the support of surrounding villagers, accused one Roger Oldrich of throwing her into the river, presumably to determine if she was a witch. The court found against Oldrich. No mention is made of Margery's husband. It would seem that she lived alone and, at least in the Oldrich case, had the support of members of the community.[44]

The apparent criminality of the ordinary medical practitioners ought not to be exaggerated: not every reference is to involvement in litigation. Religious houses and cathedrals kept detailed records of their expenses and often paid independent medical practitioners for their medicines and services. This is a constant feature of such records throughout the later medieval period, although the summoning of a physician from outside the monastery is more frequently encountered later on.[45] Nuns also seem to have employed physicians from outside. One set of rules for the nuns of Syon stipulated that the infirmaress tend to the bodily needs of the sick according to the advice of physicians.[46] The treasurers' accounts of St. Augustine's Abbey in Canterbury from 1468 to 1469 record the payment of £7 to a certain Charles the physician, while Master John, *medicus*, was paid £5 8s. 10d. for his services and for medicines purchased for the brothers.[47] The abbey also had its own infirmarer, Brother John Assher, who was reimbursed for his expenses in the same time period.[48] In the rolls of the infirmarer of Westminster Abbey in London, John de Walcote, *medicus*, was given an annual stipend of 53s. 4d. for the year 1347–48. He held the title *medicus conventus* (religious house medic).[49] The same infirmarer's accounts record the payment of 3s. 4d. to Master John Bunne in 1393–94 for coming to the abbey to attend Brother John Stowe.[50] The abbey also called in surgeons. John Bradmore was paid 6s. 9d. for performing surgery on a certain Brother William Asshwell in 1402.[51] Master Marck, a Norwich physician, was paid 13s. 4d. for inspecting urine and 6s. 8d. for enemas and other duties about 1429, as recorded in the accounts of the Cathedral Priory of Holy Trinity, Norwich.[52] The account rolls of the abbey of Durham record the payment of 40s. to a Dominican *medicus* living in York in the late 1420s.[53]

Wills are a very useful source for the nature of the medical practitioner and give some insight into matters such as families practicing medicine together. The will of Thomas, surgeon of London, who flourished in the third quarter of the thirteenth century, shows him to have been a man of considerable property, owning several houses that he left to his wife Cecelia. Also mentioned in his will were a son, William, and daughters Katherine and Avice.[54] In another document, a quitclaim on some London tenements, William and Katherine are both called surgeons, suggesting that at least two of Thomas's children followed him in surgical practice.[55]

Two sisters and a brother practicing medicine together at the beginning of the thirteenth century were Solicita, Matilda, and John, who lived in Hertfordshire. We know of them only through their property transfers, which demonstrate considerable wealth. Solicita had a husband, William of Ford, whereas Matilda confirmed legal instruments with her own seal. John was called *medicus* in documents; Solicita and Matilda were referred to as *medica*.[56]

Much less commonly recorded than brother-sister medical teams were husband-wife associations in medical practice, but this may only reflect the accidental way such information is preserved. Certainly such collaborations were common in other trades.[57] One example of a team of spousal practitioners is Thomas de Rasyn and his wife, Pernell, who practiced together in Devonshire in the middle of the fourteenth century. They were accused and subsequently pardoned in the wrongful death of one of their patients, a miller named John Panyers.[58]

The most commonly documented family relationships are medical practices shared by brothers or by father and son. For instance, the London Eyre of 1276 recorded that Master John of Hexham and his brother Master Semann were arrested and thrown into Newgate Prison, suspected in the killing of Andrew le Sarazin and his valet, Richard de Langeley. Andrew, suffering from a fever, was sent some pills by Master John. Andrew and the valet, who was given the pills to keep, ate such a quantity of them that they died. The brothers eventually were acquitted.[59] A father-son team of *medici* were John of Wakefield and his son, also called John, who flourished in the first years of the fourteenth century.[60]

Very much like the familial relationship was that between master and apprentice. Apprentices entered into a master craftsman's household for a fee and were taught a trade.[61] Medieval records give little information about the apprentice-master relationship in the medical trades, and most of that is from London rather than outlying areas.[62] For instance, London surgeon Nicholas Bradmore sued Richard Asser, a Southwark barber, in 1405, charging the barber with leaving Nicholas's service before the end of his contract. Richard countersued Nicholas and his relative John Bradmore in 1406.[63] There are rather more records of masters mentioning apprentices in their wills, and they are often treated as sons. London surgeon Henry Assheborne, in a will drawn up in 1442, gave a number of surgical books to his son, also named Henry; to his apprentice John Bolton, he left a silver belt and a furred gown.[64] John Wright, apprentice to the London surgeon Robert Braunche, was treated even more generously. In 1458 he was willed hooded gowns, cash, a silver box, and all of Robert's medicines and surgical instruments.[65] The redoubtable London surgeon Thomas Morstede was left books on medicine and surgery by his master Thomas Dayron in 1407. Morstede was executor of Dayron's will in partnership with Dayron's wife, Isabella.[66] Thomas in turn left his apprentice Robert Brynard instruments, money, silver, and a book in English in 1450.[67]

It is possible to document more detailed family relationships among medical tradespeople and even mobility between the status of tradesperson and the status of elite practitioner toward the end of the fifteenth century. London surgeon John Hobbes in 1463 willed the bulk of his estate to his son William, also a surgeon, and John's widow, Juliana. John left his apprentice John Northone a metal bowl and a copper pot. He also mentioned the forgiveness of a debt owed to him and to one John Dagvyle, probably the surgeon, who was in turn the father of another London surgeon also called John.[68] The elder Dagvyle was involved in numerous gifts of properties and loans, some to his fellow surgeons, revealing an intricate web of obligation among members of his trade.[69]

John Hobbes also directed in his will that his books, including "my book called Guido"—presumably a copy of the popular surgery of Montpellier surgeon Guy de Chauliac—be sold to cover his funeral expenses.[70] Interestingly, the younger John Dagvyle also willed two books called "Guydo" in 1487, the shorter to fellow surgeon John Hert and the longer to the London Fellowship of Surgeons.[71] William Hobbes, the son of John, moved up through the ranks of the London Barbers' Company, studied medicine at both Oxford and Cambridge, and held positions at various times as royal surgeon and royal physician. His military service as a physician and surgeon was extensive.[72]

ELITE CLERICAL PRACTITIONERS

Medieval records provide much more evidence for the lives of elite medical practitioners than they do for the middling variety, whose careers can be described only anecdotally and whose characteristics, as judged from what the records tell us, seem to change little during the later medieval period. The institutions of court, church, and university, much more than the nature of commercial life, shaped the lives of elite practitioners, and throughout the late medieval period, we can see how the text-based medicine they practiced became increasingly separated from other types of text-based learning.

The performance of healing as part of clerical duty in England is as old as written records. The healing miracles of Christ were of course very much a part of a ministry, and the holy included medical care in their own ministry too. The Venerable Bede, who died in 735, reported that he knew a man who knew a certain Northumbrian bishop John who taught a mute man to speak, and then aided a *medicus* in curing a skin disease on the man's head with his prayers.[73] Subsequently, the same bishop was staying at a nunnery and was told of one of the nuns, who, after a bloodletting, became grievously ill from an inflammation of her arm at the site of the bloodletting. The bishop inquired as to when the bleeding had taken place and was told it happened the fourth day after the new moon. He admonished the nuns that the bleeding had been done at the wrong time, citing a certain archbishop Theodore, who warned against bloodletting during the waxing of the moon and when the tides were rising (the moon was believed to rule both the tides and the blood). After much entreaty by the girl's mother, who was the abbess, the reluctant bishop agreed to see the girl, and healed her wound, thus enabling her to praise the Lord.[74]

The lives of holy men and women were considerably less fraught with healing miracles after the Norman Conquest in 1066 than they had been in the glory days of Christian missionizing about which Bede wrote. And yet considerable medical learning might still be expected in a person of notable piety. Master Ralph, *medicus*, a canon of Lincoln who flourished in the middle of the twelfth century, left no medical books to the cathedral, but only those of religious interest.[75] Probably the most celebrated clerical medical practitioner of the late eleventh and early twelfth centuries was the Tuscan churchman Faritius, who died in 1117. Faritius first came from Italy to England as cellarer of Malmesbury Abbey in Wiltshire.[76] In 1100 he was named abbot of Abingdon, near Oxford.[77] Faritius distinguished himself as a biographer of the Anglo-Saxon saint Aldhelm, noting that the Evangelist Luke was, like himself, a physician.[78] In 1101 a reason for his ecclesiastical preferment was revealed when he was summoned to attend Queen Matilda at the birth of her first child, to extend care and to interpret prognostications ("curam impendere, prognostica edicere").[79] That the queen's child died in infancy seems not to have discredited the abbot in royal eyes. Faritius continued to attend the queen in childbirth, and she never failed to patronize him, as did many others.[80] His prowess as a physician was such that Henry I trusted him alone to prepare his medicine.[81] Faritius's textual learning no doubt served him in good stead to offer explanations for unfortunate medical outcomes, especially the death of a child. His chronicler provided numerous examples of noble patrons who trusted him, as did Queen Matilda, even when their loved ones died. In one case, he gained for the abbey a generous gift of lands from the family of a little boy who perished under the abbot's care. His chronicler was probably echoing Faritius's words of comfort when he noted about the inevitable tragic outcome "there is no medicine for death."[82]

Faritius distinguished himself in rebuilding and expanding the abbey, in acquiring gifts for it from his wealthy patrons, and in having books copied for the abbey library, including many on medicine ("multos libros de physica").[83] He was a formidable feudal landlord, a shrewd lawyer, a collector of relics, and a copious correspondent on theological matters. Faritius was also praised for being a witty raconteur, and for founding a grammar school.[84] The nature of his medical training was not recorded. Some have suggested Salerno, but other than his being Italian, there is no evidence for this. He need not have studied medicine or any other subject at a university, and one assumes that his medical knowledge was acquired as a part of general knowledge in a monastic school.[85] Faritius seems to have used his learning to acquire money for the abbey. For him, and for others, it would seem, medicine was an important tool for gaining patronage.

Faritius suffered from attacks leveled at many clerical practitioners throughout the medieval period. First of all, he was criticized for being a foreigner,[86] as were many physicians and churchmen of his time and after. Second, he was attacked for his luxury. It was said that he had a separate dining hall built at the abbey for himself, in which the food was superior to that served to the other monks. The abbey was said to be filled with lavish tapestries and recherché relics, and the abbot was criticized as a stay-at-home, who neglected to attend the proper meetings and assemblies.[87] The crowning blow came in 1114 when Henry I, husband of Queen Matilda, attempted to nominate Faritius to replace his fellow Italian, Anselm, as archbishop of Canterbury. However, the powerful bishops Roger of Salisbury and Robert Bloet of Lincoln objected that a man who had devoted himself so assiduously to the examination of women's urine ought not become archbishop.[88] This account by the anonymous Abingdon chronicler differs markedly from that offered by William of Malmesbury, who characteristically blamed Faritius's foreign origins, not his medical practice, for the failure of Faritius's candidacy.[89] The actual reasons for the failure were doubtless more political than medical, but the fact remains that medical practitioners like Faritius—foreigners who consorted with women—were open to such attacks.

John of Cella, abbot of St. Albans in Hertford, who died in 1214, had a life in some ways similar to that of Faritius a century earlier. But John did not make the mistake of being a foreigner, looking at women's urine, or amassing wealth either for himself or for his abbey. John came from Bedfordshire and was educated in Paris.[90] Like so many of his fellow clerical physicians, he was educationally a man of parts: "In grammar a Priscian, in verse an Ovid, and in medicine he could be judged a Galen," the St. Albans chronicler said of him.[91] He became abbot in 1195 and engaged in a largely unsuccessful rebuilding program, all the while fighting the claims of his neighbor Robert Fitz-Walter to encroach on the abbey's properties.[92] Unlike Faritius or his medical associate Grimbald, John of Cella practiced his medicine on fellow monks, not on outside patrons. He predicted his death by uroscopy three days in advance, which gave him time to prepare for death, an important precaution to ensure safe passage of his soul. Such a feat of uroscopic virtuosity could not have failed to impress: his chronicler referred to John as an "outstanding physician, and an incomparable judge of urines." John apologized to his brothers for his sins, kissed them good-bye, was anointed ("oleo sancto infirmorum est inunctus"), and retired to his chamber to die. Since the abbot was partly blind at the time, his uroscopic prophecy had to be confirmed by fellow monk Master William of Bedford.[93]

Men like John of Cella, Faritius, and Bede's bishop John have a shaky claim to the title of medical practitioner. They were instead holy men, whose lives were written down in part as a lesson in piety to others. Part of their holiness was the performance of healing duties, but more important, these men offered explanations for medical phenomena that were based on rationality and learning. They reasoned why something had happened, or would happen, suggesting explanations based on an understanding of the natural world. Learned medicine was, for them and for their audiences, a useful way of imposing some sort of rational order on the spectacle of disease and death that confronted them. For these people, nothing happened by chance: a learned and holy man could reveal the true causes of seemingly meaningless events and, thus, the design of God that lay behind them.

During the early thirteenth century in England, the centers of text-based medical learning shifted from monastic settings to the new universities of Oxford and Cambridge. Oftentimes a learned physician would have studied in several different places, for there were flourishing universities in France and Italy boasting famous teachers, and medieval students often traveled widely. Nicholas of Farnham, for example, studied and taught at Paris, Bologna, Cambridge, and Oxford during the first half of the thirteenth century and performed various diplomatic offices, as well as serving as royal physician to Henry III and Queen Eleanor.[94] As early as 1223 he was paid for drugs and electuaries (medicinal pastes) supplied to the king. He also seems to have seen patients of a less august ranking. In 1239 he received 40s. for the treatment of Roger le Panetiere, who lay sick at Woodstock.[95] Nicholas's income was supplemented considerably from 1219 by permission to hold a number of benefices at the same time.[96] He became bishop of Durham in 1241, which occasioned a chronicler to remark that "a physician of bodies was made a physician of souls."[97]

Matthew Paris, the principal source for Farnham's life, portrayed his subject as a man of extraordinary modesty and wisdom, whose combination of piety and medical knowledge prompted the papal legate Otto in 1237 to advise the king and queen to employ him not only as their physician but also as their confessor.[98] In 1244, Matthew said, Farnham was relieved of an incurable jaundice by a drink made from the hairs of the beard of St. Edmund of Abingdon, a relic preserved by the saint's barber.[99] Farnham's medical degrees are not recorded, but his reputation for piety, wisdom, discretion, and, above all, good advice, seem to have been qualification enough for the king and queen, inasmuch as they used his priestly, diplomatic, and medical services.

Nicholas of Farnham was only one of several physician-bishops who flourished from the thirteenth century onward. John Dalderby, bishop of Lincoln, received his master of arts from Oxford by 1269 and his doctorate of theology by about 1290, and was said to have studied and lectured in the faculty of medicine at Oxford. Such was his reputation for sanctity that those praying at his tomb were granted an indulgence in 1321, though an attempt to have him canonized failed in 1327.[100] Hugh of Evesham, another probable student and lecturer at Oxford and Paris, was called to Rome perhaps in 1279 to answer some difficult medical questions and to give advice about a "fever" that had been raging there. He held a number of ecclesiastical incomes at once to the end of his life, and was made cardinal by his papal patron Martin IV in 1281. He died in Rome in 1287. Hugh's longer medical writings appear not to have survived, but recipes and a sermon are extant.[101]

Another physician-bishop was Tideman de Winchcombe (d. 1401), a Cistercian who attended Richard II. Richard had him appointed abbot of Beaulieu and later bishop of Llandaff. By 1396 he had progressed to the bishopric of Worcester, an honor he received in the presence of the king. His formal education is unknown, but his learning must have been considerable, for he worked not only as a successful Cistercian churchman and trusted courtier but also as a surgeon.[102]

Just as clerical practitioners practiced their medicine as a part of other duties befitting learned men, so medical writers, also clerics, for the most part wrote on medicine as a part of general knowledge. During the early part of the thirteenth century, John Blund wrote *Tractatus de anima* (Treatise on the soul), a topic that would have held medical interest for medieval thinkers.[103] Also at the beginning of the thirteenth century, Alfred of Sareshel wrote his *De motu cordis* (On the motion of the heart).[104] Both works were based on medical and Aristotelian natural philosophical texts. Neither man left the slightest evidence of medical practice, and so it is important to remember that not everyone who wrote on medicine was necessarily a medical practitioner.

Such was the case with Bartholomew the Englishman (Bartholomaeus Anglicus), who wrote a popular encyclopedia in Latin that dates from about 1250.[105] Bartholomew composed his work, *De proprietatibus rerum* (On the properties of things), as a guide to the study of Holy Scripture. It covers such diverse topics as the number of angels, how to select a good servant, and the variety of plants and animals and their moral characteristics. It also includes a chapter on medicine based on the writings of the Italian monk Constantine the African.[106] Once again, there is no evidence that Bartholomew ever practiced medicine. For him, a knowledge of medicine was part of a general encyclopedic knowledge of the created universe.

The so-called rise of universities, the institutionalization of the learning that surrounded new translations of Aristotle from Arabic into Latin, added another framework to that of court and church in which the physician could establish himself. English universities were founded on older Continental models, and English-educated medical doctors cannot be found until the fourteenth century. Before that, Englishmen studied abroad, many times returning to England, like Nicholas of Farnham, to serve in the church and at court. Still others studied medicine at university without proceeding to a degree.[107]

Several prominent medical figures seem to have never formed a definite association with a university, and no doubt this arrangement should be regarded as very common in the learned world. The Anglo-Norman physician and cleric Gilbert Eagle (Gilbertus Anglicus) had several prominent English patrons, and appeared as witness with other English physicians in legal documents. There is no certain evidence he studied medicine at any university, although his medical learning was unparalleled for his time in England.[108] A similar educational-related obscurity surrounds the prolific Latin medical writer Richard of England (Richardus Anglicus), Gilbert's near contemporary, who probably was part of a medical circle at the papal court.[109]

The universities of Oxford and Cambridge, with medical faculties dating from the later thirteenth century, became from that time increasingly powerful institutional forces in the lives of elite English medical practitioners. From the early fourteenth century, these universities began to grant their own medical degrees, allowing English physicians to study, form alliances, and find employment at home. Oxford master Roger Fabell, for instance, was appointed to teach grammar to the novices at Oseney Abbey in the mid-fifteenth century. Like the more august clerical figures discussed above, Roger performed a number of functions. He taught, served as chaplain, and acted as physician to the abbey.[110]

Many of these university-educated physicians demonstrated their greatest loyalty to the college at which they had been educated.[111] Stephen of Cornwall, a master of Balliol College, Oxford, in the early fourteenth century, received his medical doctorate at Paris, but left to his Balliol colleague Simon of Holbeche a manuscript containing Latin translations of Galen's writings (now Balliol College MS 231), which Simon in turn donated to the college on his death. Simon also left a copy of Serapion's *De simplicibus medicinis* (On uncompounded medicines) to Walter de Barton, rector of Dry Drayton, Cambridgeshire, whom he had known at Peterhouse, in 1335. Simon left directions that Walter in turn pass it on to Peterhouse, Cambridge. This Walter did, and the manuscript is now Peterhouse MS 140.[112]

The royal physician and clergyman Nicholas Colnet was another Oxford student, who accompanied Henry V as his doctor to Agincourt in France in 1415. The exact nature of his medical education was unknown, but Nicholas did leave a considerable fortune to his sister, brother, and a niece. Most important, he left a copy of Montpellier physician Bernard Gordon's *Lilium medicinae* (Lily of medicine) in 1420 to John Mayhew, who like Nicholas was a fellow of Merton College, Oxford, which was notable for its physicians and natural philosophers.[113] A similar loyalty was shown by the New College, Oxford, medical doctor Thomas Boket, who was active as a scholar in the middle of the fifteenth century. Thomas gave some medical texts to his college, which are in New College MS 168.[114]

Very little is known about the social origins of educated physicians in medieval England before the fifteenth century. In the early fourteenth century, John of Cobham, who held a medical doctorate from Oxford, could claim a prominent family connection: he was the bastard son of a certain Ralph of Cobham, knight. His family background is known only because of the record of exceptions that had to be made to provide him an income from the church in spite of his illegitimacy.[115] Nicholas Colnet, the Merton physician who died in 1420, was related to the founder of that college, but such information about learned English physicians before about 1425 is very rare.[116] What little evidence remains about the social backgrounds of English students in general suggests that personal connections like those of Nicholas were important to obtain support for a university education, but that very few of these students came from the upper classes.[117]

The later fifteenth century provides more information about the social standing of educated medical practitioners. Cambridge-educated physician, astronomer, and mathematician Lewis Caerleon was made a knight of the king's alms in 1488 by Henry VII, probably less in recognition of his service as physician to the king and his family and more for his assistance in intrigue against Richard III.[118] Another medical practitioner who received a knighthood was Cambridge-educated medical doctor Sir James Frise, who served Edward IV as royal physician in the later fifteenth century.[119]

The fifteenth century also saw the entry of men of high social status into the ranks of the medically educated. Several educated physicians seem to have come from wealthy families, or to have accumulated sizable fortunes for themselves. John Arundel was a medical doctor from a prominent Cornwall family who was first associated with Exeter College, Oxford. John was called physician and chaplain to Henry VI in 1454, and served the king as a diplomat in 1457. He became bishop of Chichester in 1459.[120] John Faceby, an Oxford medical doctor from Southwark, was associated with Arundel as royal physician, and managed to gain enormous royal preferments for himself, his wife, Alice, and his son, also called John.[121]

Faceby was not the only married man among university-educated physicians in the later Middle Ages. John Somerset, who held a medical doctorate, probably from Cambridge, married twice and was, like Faceby and Arunudel, physician to Henry VI. He was master of the grammar school of Bury St. Edmunds, chancellor of the exchequer, warden of the royal mint, and the donor—as well as perhaps the author—of several medical books.[122] Gilbert Kymer, the Oxford medical doctor, was said to have taken a wife, although he apparently abandoned her to become a priest and successful courtier to Humfrey, duke of Gloucester.[123]

CONCLUSION

Functionalist descriptions of medieval English medical practitioners—barber, physician, or surgeon, for example—are of limited utility in understanding the variety of duties a medical practitioner could perform. Brewers who practiced surgery, abbots who delivered babies, friars who wrote medical books, a chancellor of the exchequer who doctored the king, a Cistercian surgeon: all were involved in healing, and all were involved in other pursuits. The institutions of court, church, municipality, university, guild, and hospital that worked to separate medical practice from other duties, and medical knowledge from other forms of dignified learning, had barely begun to exert an influence in medieval England. Sufferers could seek healing from numerous kinds of people, and the choices were not obvious. Medical expertise was only beginning to distinguish itself from other abilities, making the picture of medieval English medical practice complex indeed.

CHAPTER II

Medical Travelers to England and the English Medical Practitioner Abroad

IN 1264 THE streets of London were torn by murderous riots. Although these insurrections are usually characterized as anti-Semitic, they were also directed against the Italians and French, who fled with the Jews for refuge to the Tower of London.[1] More than a century and a half later, the London mob attacked Dutch breweries, enraged by the rumor that foreigners were selling poison beer.[2] The causes of such disturbances, then and now, are complex, but viewed from a historical distance, these riots point to the fact that some residents obviously were viewed as outsiders, even though, like the Jews, they could be native-born. "Foreignness," during a time before the development of modern notions of the nation-state, is difficult to define in useful terms, especially on the island of Britain. Although isolated from the European continent geographically, Britain was bound especially to France and Italy by the institutions of court and church. Even the Anglo-Saxons had been invaders to the island, and they were followed by the Norman French in the eleventh century, who brought with them a French-speaking court, their own doctors, a Jewish community including medical practitioners, and a complicated web of relationships that kept them at turns in alliance or conflict with their French relatives. The papacy had sent missionaries to Britain since before the time of the Venerable Bede, and it retained its influence through the church from Rome and, during the fourteenth century, from its seat in Avignon in the south of France. Christian clerics could communicate with each other in western Europe's universal tongue—Latin—which contributed to professional and geographical mobility, at least among the educated. Trade added to the presence of foreigners during the later Middle Ages, for England distinguished itself as a center of commerce, maintaining contact with the Continent and the Mediterranean world through its port cities.

Commerce, family alliances, warfare, and church affairs all assured that, among other visitors to the island, foreign doctors would be a constant feature of the English medical scene, and ensured that opportunities for foreign travel were available to English medical practitioners as well. Foreigners excited ill feelings among the English at many levels of society, especially when they were seen to be usurping favors from the natives. Jews experienced anti-Semitism, even when they were native-born. Nevertheless, foreigners and foreign travel were facts of life for a large number of English medical practitioners and for their patrons. More important, foreign contact made certain that English medicine was shaped by non-English trade and learning.

THE CASE OF THE JEWISH COMMUNITIES

The first Jewish settlement in England was in London and was made up by and large of Jews who had followed William the Conqueror from France in 1066, coming to England for the commercial opportunities residence there could offer. Like William, his followers, and his descendants, these Jews transacted legal and commercial business in French. Of course, they used Hebrew among themselves, and many no doubt could understand Latin.[3] There is some suggestion that learned English Jews were familiar with English, Aramaic, and Arabic.[4] The medieval Jewish community attained a high level of literacy, at least among the socially elite. Jews were almost always confined to their own groups, which spread from London to important provincial cities like York, Norwich, Canterbury, the university towns of Oxford and Cambridge, and elsewhere,[5] especially during the anarchy of the reign of King Stephen (1135–1154).[6] Different from most English people linguistically, religiously, ethnically, and in their diet, Jews always remained at the mercy of the ruling Christians and never gained the rights of citizenship granted to gentiles.[7]

Jews were limited in the trades they could pursue—most were involved in money-lending—which made them useful to the cash-hungry nobility who were almost always at war. Usury—charging interest for use of money—was technically forbidden to Christians,[8] but the lack of rigor with which this prohibition was observed has only recently been appreciated.[9] The Crusades more than anything motivated the papacy to wink at usury among Christians, and Jews were even coerced by Rome to loan money to crusaders.[10] Jewish and Christian establishments were in conflict with each other over money-lending,[11] for the Jewish community held superior expertise, as well as cash, in a society whose trade was based in large part on barter—which no doubt led them to England in the first place.[12] Jews not only lent money; they also dealt in commercial affairs that reflected their networks of kinship and obligation on the European continent. Their legal affairs were recorded in what is called the Exchequer of the Jews, a sort of government "Department of Jewish Affairs," as one historian has put it.[13]

Jews were tolerated in England not only as a source of credit but also as a source of revenue. Their function as moneylenders was increasingly usurped by Christians, most notably by Queen Eleanor of Provence, widow of Henry III and mother of Edward I, who confiscated much of their wealth and had them expelled from her dower towns in 1275.[14] Jews were singled out for taxation, prosecution, fines, and execution at a much higher rate than their Christian counterparts.[15] There is evidence in England that Jews were forced to attend Christian conversion sermons by 1280.[16] The anti-Semitism that lay behind this treatment, always present among English churchmen[17] but exacerbated by the new orders of friars at the end of the thirteenth century,[18] allowed much of Jews' wealth to be confiscated at their expulsion from England in 1290. Their numbers then in all of England may have been between 2,500 and 3,000.[19] Many returned to France, and a year later were forced from there by Philip.[20] After the expulsion, Jews were found occasionally in England, but needed special license to enter, for example, to give medical treatment to a Christian patron.[21]

The role of the Jewish physician in England is less well understood than that of his gentile counterpart, no doubt due to the relatively small amount of remaining evidence.[22] For instance, in 1239 the London Jewish medical practitioner Milo was assessed 2s. 5d. in tax, tying him for fifty-sixth place among ninety other Jews listed.[23] Apart from this tantalizing hint, no more about Milo is known. Rarely, there is a bit more to go on. What little information remains points to the fact that Jewish and Christian physicians resembled each other in several ways. Like many Christian practitioners, the rabbi, or teacher, combined medical advice with other kinds of learned advice that his textual study made him qualified to dispense.[24] Medical learning may have taken place in the synagogue (in Latin *scola Iudeorum* or school of the Jews) along with other types of textual learning, but in England this topic has yet to be explored.[25] Quite a bit is known, however, about Jewish men of high social standing in England. For instance, Rabbi Elijah Menahem ben Rabbi Moses (in Latin, Magister Elias fil' Magistri Mossei), who lived in London during the thirteenth century, was a notable physician to both gentiles and Jews.[26] Additionally, he was a celebrated lawyer, whose opinions on Jewish law were cited by at least one Continental legal scholar, Mordecai ben Hillel of Nuremberg.[27] Moreover, Elijah was a wealthy businessman, whose trading connections with Flanders were in grain and wool.[28] He loaned money throughout England.[29] When Elijah died, he left a wife and five sons, as well as an estate that showed him to have been a remarkably rich man. His wife, Floria, handled her own legal affairs after his death.[30]

Also, it was doubtless true in England, as it was on the Continent, that medical learning was passed down in Jewish families from father to son,[31] as it sometimes had been in Christian families. For example, during the middle of the thirteenth century, one Isaac, a rabbi and physician, practiced medicine in Norwich with his son Solomon, who owned a medicinal herb garden in that city.[32] In contrast to practice in the Christian world, however, Jews were forbidden to attend the English universities in Oxford and Cambridge, even though these towns had sizable Jewish populations serving students in need of credit.[33] Denial of the sort of medical education available to Christian men must have reinforced the practice of passing down medical knowledge from parent to child or from master to apprentice among Jews.[34]

Almost all Jewish medical practitioners known in England were physicians rather than surgeons, and although documentary evidence shows Jewish women engaged in monetary transactions such as paying taxes,[35] there are no instances of Jewish women practicing medicine in England yet known. This was not the case with Christian practitioners. Most data about English surgical practitioners is found in connection with their membership in trade guilds, which were Christian organizations, and this no doubt militates against the survival of records of Jewish surgical practice. One exception is the London surgeon (*le cyrurgien*) Sampson, who mainperned (bailed out) a fellow Jew in 1273, but his status as a surgeon is mentioned only in passing.[36]

Jewish physicians were known to have practiced among gentiles (although we have no information that the opposite was true). Many were accomplished scholars, who held the advantage over their Christian counterparts of being able to read medical texts in Arabic and Hebrew, a talent nearly lost in the Latin-speaking West.[37] The monk and chronicler William of Newburgh lamented the murder of an unnamed Jewish physician of Lynn, in Norfolk, by an anti-Semitic mob in 1190. William noted that the unfortunate physician was well thought of in the Christian community because of his good character and medical skill.[38] The aforementioned Elijah, physician, merchant, and rabbi of London, was called upon in 1280 to attend Jean d'Avesnes, a nephew of the count of Flanders, lying ill probably in Valenciennes (in Flanders), where the doctor had trading connections. According to a petition he sent in French to Chancellor Robert Burnell asking safe conduct, he had recommended treatment for Jean by letter. Elijah wanted to treat the nephew in person, "for a man can do better by sight than by hearsay" [kar um put myues ouere par vewe ke par oye].[39] Henry I may have been treated by the famous Jewish convert Petrus Alfonsi (Moses Sephardi), a remarkably accomplished Andalusian scholar who was baptized in 1106.[40]

Even after the Jews were forced to flee in 1290, their activities as medical practitioners in England continued. Some came as converts, but others, such as the French Jew Samson de Mierbeawe (Sansone di Mirebello), who was called to attend Alice Fitzwaryn, wife of the famous lord mayor of London Richard Whittington, in 1409, obtained special license to practice their faith while attending a powerful patron.[41] At about the same time the

Jewish physician of Bologna Elias Sabot (Elijah ben Shabbetai) received permission to attend Henry IV in England. Elias was professor at Padua and had popes and noblemen, among his Italian medical patrons, one of whom granted him a knighthood.[42]

FOREIGN MEDICAL PRACTITIONERS IN ENGLAND

The issue of who was a foreigner in England became important only toward the end of the medieval period. Churchmen (many of whom were physicians), the nobility, and members of their retinues (also often physicians) were seldom subject to questions of national origin. In a feudal society, where loyalty was to a person and not to land or country, the question of citizenship was hardly important. When the issue was raised, the assurance of a person's native birth was sufficient. Two interrelated factors—the Hundred Years' War (1337–1453) and the growth of trade with the Continent in the fourteenth century—worked to make necessary refinements in legal definitions of Englishness. The development of taxes on trade, rather than on land, and issues raised by the claims of English monarchs to French territories led to parliamentary distinctions of the definition of citizenship that affected foreigners in general and foreign medical practitioners in particular.[43]

The English crown held disputed lands in France and depended on loyalty from people there, especially in Gascony, which supported the lucrative wine trade. The birth of children to English parents in France raised problems of citizenship, and legal residence in England could be used as a reward for loyal service to the king in time of war.[44] The need by the Crown for revenue to supply its war efforts in France made taxation of exports by foreigners attractive.[45] Definition of a resident's precise legal status could make the difference between heavy taxation and immunity, and between access to law courts and denial of justice, so Parliament was forced to develop useful means of granting legal residence. By the fifteenth century, even the nobility made sure to obtain English legal status.[46]

England's nearest neighbor on the Continent, both geographically and culturally, was France. Not surprisingly, French physicians formed the bulk of foreign practitioners before the fifteenth century in England.[47] Like Jewish physicians, the lives of these foreign physicians can best be understood in relationship to the careers of their patrons and to the political and social conditions under which they lived. Little about ordinary French medical practitioners in England (if they existed in any number at all) is known: almost all the information that survives concerns elite clerical practitioners. French physicians were known in England even before the Norman Conquest.[48] Baldwin, born in the famous cathedral and school city of

Chartres, was brought to England to attend Edward the Confessor, the last Anglo-Saxon king, in 1059. He later attended William the Conqueror and Lanfranc, archbishop of Canterbury. Although active as a physician, Baldwin also participated in church affairs, settling disputes in Rome and becoming a celebrated abbot of Bury St. Edmunds.[49]

The conquest brought a new French court to England, which contained learned physicians. William the Conqueror established his claim to the English throne by force of arms in 1066. He was attended by a fellow Norman, the physician Gilbert Maminot, the son of a knight and himself bishop of Lisieux, east of Caen.[50] Like so many learned medical practitioners of his time, Gilbert served William as a physician and chaplain,[51] and probably attended his wife, Queen Matilda.[52] In addition to medical services, Gilbert represented his patron on church business in Rome.[53] He was present at the death of William after a riding accident in Rouen in 1087, and along with other physicians predicted William's death by means of uroscopy.[54] Gilbert's chronicler and younger acquaintance Orderic Vitalis portrayed his ecclesiastical patron as a man with virtues and vices like those of the Italian physician Faritius: learning, eloquence, wealth, and luxury. He was a notable teacher of the liberal arts, especially astronomy, and loved many of the diversions his father must have allowed him as a boy: gambling, hunting, and other mundane pursuits.[55] Gilbert died in 1101.[56] Orderic, although he lived in Normandy, was English-born, and expressed an Englishman's distaste for what he saw as the flashy, foreign, and self-indulgent ways of the French, just as close contemporary William of Malmesbury had for other foreigners.[57]

Family connections and landholdings suggest that Gilbert must have spent time in England, but this is conjectural. We can be more certain in that respect about Gilbert's near contemporary John of Villula, also called John of Tours from his birthplace in France. John attended William the Conqueror in his last illness along with Gilbert. He became bishop of Wells through the patronage of William's son, William Rufus, who made him royal chaplain in 1087 and bishop a year later.[58] John too fell under the critical eye of William of Malmesbury, who found his medical knowledge rather too practical, and his devotion to literature and the finer things in life unsettling.[59] The seduction of the medicinal waters at the nearby city of Bath led the new bishop to move his seat there in 1090.[60] Having used his medical skills, rude though they may have been, to attract royal patronage, John seems to have given up his medical practice altogether on becoming bishop. He died in 1122.[61]

The Crusades, in which Christians fought to regain the Holy Lands from the Muslims, occupied the attention of English monarchs and their medical retinues through much of the twelfth century. Richard I, son of Henry II, spent very little time in England, preferring a life of adventure on the

Continent. Richard seems to have been accompanied by one Malger (Mauger), probably of French birth, who is variously called king's *medicus* and *clericus* (clerk) by chroniclers.[62] He was not at his master's side when Richard received his fatal wound during a siege in Poitou in 1199, having returned to England to be named bishop of Worcester. Richard was attended by an unnamed surgeon instead.[63] Supporting the papal interdict against Richard's brother King John in 1208, Malger fled to France and died there in 1212.[64] Like John of Villula, Malger seems to have abandoned medical practice on his elevation to a bishopric.

Peter of Joinzac came from modern-day Jonzac, north of Bordeaux. He was physician to John's son Henry III from 1235–1255 and followed Henry to France in 1242. Peter received numerous royal and ecclesiastical incomes from the king's patronage, both in England and in Bordeaux.[65] William of Fécamp, from northwest of Rouen, had a similar career to that of Malger. He began as clerk of Henry III's brother Richard, and was Henry's physician by 1263. From that time onward, he received numerous incomes from the church and from royal gifts.[66]

Henry married Eleanor of Provence in 1236, and she brought her medical practitioners to England with her. Peter de Alpibus was referred to in a letter from Adam Marsh to Robert Grosseteste in 1251 as the queen's *medicus*, and as a learned man of great probity. His ecclesiastical incomes at the queen's patronage were considerable.[67] Henry and Eleanor were also attended by the Englishman Nicholas of Farnham, one of the first physicians educated at Oxford, who was professor of medicine at the University of Bologna and later bishop of Durham. He was more of a diplomat than a medical practitioner, however, and seems to have acted to smooth delicate relations with the papal curia.[68]

The growth of the medical faculties at Oxford and Cambridge during the fourteenth century increasingly supplied royal and noble households with a native source of learned practitioners. Moreover, the Hundred Years' War understandably made life more complicated for French doctors who wanted to attach themselves to wealthy patrons. But the French physician did not disappear from the English scene altogether. William Radicis, a priest and Paris-educated physician, attended his master, the French monarch John II, during his captivity in London from 1357 to 1360, returning to France on occasion to bring back entertaining romances for the exiled king to read.[69] Henry IV, whose adventures included a crusade to Lithuania and wars at home and abroad, had as one of his physicians Louis Recouches, whose name indicates a French origin. In spite of—or perhaps because of—his foreign origins, he was given the lucrative office of keeper of the Tower mint in 1406.[70] This office he turned over to another royal physician and foreigner, the Italian David de Nigarellis de Lucca, in 1408.[71] By 1439 an English physician, Cambridge M.D. John Somerset, held the same post at the behest of Henry VI.[72] Henry IV's third son, John, duke of Bedford, who caused Joan of Arc to be burned as a witch in 1431, was attended in his extensive French travels by Philibert Fournier, a Paris-educated physician. Philibert may have followed his master to London in 1433, and probably attended him at his death at Rouen in 1435.[73]

Records of French physicians not attached to a royal or noble person are rare in medieval England. Burgundian John of Auence had practiced in London for several years before attempting to return to the Continent with his wife, Mary, in 1362, citing his neighbors' hostility to foreigners. His belongings were seized on the way to Flanders and were returned only on appeal of Edward III.[74] The doctor's ability to obtain royal intercession perhaps indicates important patronage not elsewhere recorded.

French surgeons are not noticed as often as physicians, but appeared in royal households from the late thirteenth century. Simon of Beauvais was surgeon to Edward I and amassed a considerable fortune from royal favor, which he passed on to his son Philip, who followed his father in the king's service. Simon attended other patients in London, and at Marlborough in the late 1270s. Records survive of his expenses.[75] Philip, also a married man, followed Edward I in his campaigns in Gascony in 1297, apparently in the capacity of a military surgeon. He may have had a brother, Simon, who was an English parson.[76] Surgeon Martin de Vere was in royal service in France perhaps as late as 1348. From his master he obtained a number of favors, including pardon for a murder and subsequent banishment from Bayonne (near Biarritz), assistance against the citizens of Bordeaux, and a new horse in 1313. He may never have been in England.[77] Stephen of Paris was another surgeon to Edward II, in charge of providing medical supplies to the royal army in Scotland. Apart from his name, there is no other evidence of his French origins.[78] Finally, a letter of denization in 1443 identified Michael Belwell as a Frenchman, and a yeoman and surgeon to Henry VI.[79]

Unlike the French, who became less numerous in England toward the end of the medieval period, Italian medical practitioners increased in number and influence. French doctors are most in evidence as clerics who attached themselves to a royal or noble person who was herself or himself French, or who was resident for some time in French-speaking lands. Italians, by contrast, came to England for the most part as entrepreneurs. Some, especially under the Normans and early Plantagenets, were, like Faritius and Grimbald, sent to England by their monastic orders as professional administrators. Most, however, came of their own accord, pursuing the typical Italian callings of money-lending, sea trade, and the search for patronage.

The expulsion of the Jews at the end of the thirteenth century marked a transfer from money-lending controlled by Jewish families to credit controlled by Italian banking concerns. The great banking houses of the Ricci-

ardi, Frescobaldi, Bardi, and Peruzzi financed various royal military campaigns and in return gained immunities and preferments that allowed
them to control many types of trade, the wool trade especially.[80] Italian
medical practitioners in England during the fourteenth and fifteenth centuries resembled Jewish ones in that they often were attached to an elite
English patron, but remained very much part of a community of their con-
freres, and involved themselves in other aspects of commerce apart from
medical practice, including money-lending and commodities trading.
Some sought or obtained denization, and many used their contacts with
the Continent to their advantage in trade and banking.

Pancio da Controne was almost a stereotype of the successful Italian phy-
sician-entrepreneur in England. He came from near Lucca, northeast of
Pisa, and served as physician to Isabella of France, her husband, Edward
II, and their son, Edward III. A legal advocate for his fellow Italians in
London, former physician to the Frescobaldi family at the papal court in
Avignon, and noted authority on fevers, Pancio made considerable money
in the wool trade, an industry at the very center of English commerce. His
chief patron in this regard was Queen Isabella herself. In addition, Pancio
amassed a fortune in landholdings throughout southern England, some of
which were confiscated from Hugh Le Despenser the Younger by Queen
Isabella and given to him. In addition, he had annuities gained from his
royal patrons, whom he followed around Britain and to the Continent on
their various expeditions. His connections with the Italian banking and
trading families of Bardi and Frescobaldi seem to have served him well. In
the year of his death, 1340, Pancio had loaned Edward III the astronomical
sum of nearly six and a half thousand pounds.[81]

Scattered references to Italian physicians reveal others to have been involved in the wool trade as well as in medicine. Francisco de Massa Sancti
Petri, a London *fisicien*, obtained royal favor in a dispute with other Italians
over a wool shipment in 1327.[82] Lodowyk de Arecia, from Aricia near
Rome, was involved in 1345 in the London sale of alum, used in the pro-
cessing of wool.[83] No doubt contact with Continental business partners or
family members made many kinds of trade possible. For instance, Master
Peter Lombard, a physician who attended the monks at the Westminster
Abbey Infirmary in the early 1360s, was paid 16s. 2d. for medicines he ordered from his Lombard apothecary.[84]

Many Italian physicians seem to have maintained associations with other
Italians while in England. The Neapolitan physician Master Anthony de
Romanis was given bail in 1394 by three Florentines, and in turn posted
bail in 1407, again with three Florentines.[85] More remarkable are the records left of Italians who sought or gained English associations or residency.
Peter of Florence was in the retinues of both Edward III and Queen Philippa by 1368. He received the sum of £40 a year for his services paid from

the exchequer.[86] Pascal of Bologna, styled in various documents as a surgeon or *medicus*, was surgeon to Henry, duke of Lancaster, in the middle of the fourteenth century. Henry obtained several ecclesiastical benefices in England for Pascal from the pope. Pascal was sworn before the mayor and aldermen of the City of London in 1354 with two other London surgeons to give expert testimony in the case of possible surgical malfeasance by John the Spicer of Cornhill. Two years later he was paid £13 6s. 8d. for curing Elizabeth, countess of Ulster.[87]

Peter of Milan was another medical adventurer who came to England from Paris at the request of Richard Courtenay, bishop of Norwich, probably in 1413. He became enmeshed in a number of complex diplomatic intrigues, all the while serving as physician to several royal and noble patrons, including Joan of Navarre, Henry V, and Lucia, countess of Kent, who like Peter was a native of Lombardy.[88]

James of Milan, physician to Henry VI, petitioned the king along with another man from Milan in 1431 for permission to remain in London and set up trade there.[89] Two years later, John de Signorellis, who came to England at the request of Humfrey, duke of Gloucester, was granted denization by Parliament at the request of the king.[90]

The French and the Italians seem to have formed the dominant groups of foreign medical practitioners in medieval England, but scattered records remain of migrants from other countries. The inhabitants of the low countries and German-speaking lands, loosely characterized in documents as "Dutch," formed a significant group of aliens especially in London during the fifteenth century and afterward.[91] Records of these practitioners come late in the century, but a few are worth mention. Anthony Baldewyn, a physician from Middelburg, apparently practiced medicine in London in the parish of St. Clement's, possibly on Candlewick Street. He left a number of books in his will, which was proved in 1458, including works by Arnald of Villanova, the aphorisms of Hippocrates, the regimen of the School of Salerno, a French version of Bernard Gordon's *Lilium medicinae*, and the ninth book of Almansor. Some of those named as recipients of books in his will had Italian names.[92]

Gerard van Delft, a physician, transferred his goods to a fellow Dutchman, Paul van de Bessen, in 1458. About him no more is known.[93] James Frise, born in Friesland, was a Cambridge medical doctor and served as physician to Edward IV. He was married, and gained numerous favors from his royal patrons, including denization in 1473.[94] Another "Ducheman," James le Leche, petitioned Edward IV from prison in London, where he had been thrown by Sir Edward Courtney in a dispute about his medical fee.[95]

Medical practitioners from the Iberian Peninsula sometimes made their presence known. Peter of Portugal, *phisicus regis*, attended Edward I at the end of the thirteenth century. A letter by him survives in which he attempted to intercede with Sir John de Langeton, the chancellor, on behalf of London merchants from Portugal.[96] The cleric Peter Dalcobace came to England from Alcobaça, near Lisbon, and attended several members of the royal family. He received denization in 1420, and probably attended Joan of Navarre, second wife of Henry IV, as well as the king himself. Much of the documentation that surrounds his English career involved disputes over the ecclesiastical incomes assigned to him by the king.[97] Laurence Gomes was another Portuguese physician who, like Peter, received disputed ecclesiastical incomes from Henry IV, presumably in return for medical service. He died in 1428.[98]

Paul Gabrielis, a Spanish physician, received pensions for medical service from Edward III and Richard II. His yearly pension of £20 was established in 1376.[99] In 1392 physician John de Spayne managed to receive denization under the patronage of Richard II to pursue medical practice in London for four years.[100]

Greek physician Demetrius de Cerno was granted denization in 1424 by Parliament under Henry VI, possibly at the intercession of Lucia Visconti, countess of Kent (the Visconti of Milan had connections with England through a dynastic marriage with the family of Edward III), who remembered the doctor in her will. Demetrius argued for his residency by stating that he was married to an Englishwoman and that they had children.[101] Medical doctor Thomas Frank was probably Greek, and is principally known through disputes in the mid-fifteenth century over his ecclesiastical incomes, which opponents claimed were given to him by the pope even though he was not in holy orders. He maintained business dealings with several Venetians, including Bernard Barbo.[102]

A lone Swiss survives in the records: Master Lewis of Basel. Lewis is noticed in inventory of aliens and their worth ordered by Henry IV and made in Candlewick ward, London, in 1406. His worth was estimated at 5 marks.[103]

ENGLISH MEDICAL PRACTITIONERS ABROAD

Foreign medical practitioners came to England for patronage, wealth, and as a part of clerical duty. English people were drawn abroad for all those reasons too. But the weakness of medical faculties at Oxford and Cambridge, and the exacerbations and remissions in Continental campaigns of the Hundred Years' War added to the attractions of foreign travel for the English medical practitioner.[104] War and education were the primary seductions for the Englishman abroad, with the latter generating the most evidence of medical activity.[105]

The first medical university in the West was at Salerno, in southern Italy, which was closely associated with the Benedictine abbey of Monte Cassino, where Constantine the African had first translated basic medical texts for the use of the scholars there. Perhaps surprisingly, there is very little evidence that Englishmen studied medicine at Salerno, although there are no doubt gaps in the records. Warin, who became abbot of St. Albans and died in 1195, studied medicine at Salerno with his brother Matthew ("in physica apud Salernum eleganter atque efficaciter erudito").[106] Warin left no record of practice, and it is likely that his medical learning was part of a general education. He was followed as abbot by the physician John of Cella.[107]

The University of Bologna was a seemingly more popular magnet for medical studies for English students. Nicholas Farnham had studied medicine there, and others left records as well. Hugh, an Englishman, appears in the records of the university at the end of the thirteenth century.[108] Martin Joce had his bachelor of medicine degree from Bologna transferred at Oxford by 1476.[109]

Among other Italian universities, Padua drew several students. Cambridge's most famous physician, John Argentine, probably took his M.D. from there by 1465,[110] as did the Cambridge physician John Clerke in 1477.[111] John Free received his M.D. at about the time Argentine was granted his.[112] Another Cambridge physician granted his doctorate at Padua in the fifteenth century was William Hattecliffe, in 1447.[113]

Although not a university, the papal court in Rome during the thirteenth century also seems to have drawn clerical physicians as a center for learning in medicine and related topics.[114] The Cistercian cardinal John of Toledo attended Pope Innocent IV, who maintained a close alliance with Henry III from Rome. John was an Englishman, in spite of his mysterious name, and wrote a much copied regimen of health, *De conservanda sanitate* (On conserving health). He died in 1275.[115] Cardinal Hugh of Evesham was called from England to Rome in 1280 to consult about a fever that had been raging there. He died and was buried in Rome in 1287.[116]

Montpellier, like Salerno, seems to have attracted surprisingly few English medical students. In 1246 Henry III gave 40s. to a Richard the physician to support his study there.[117] Arnald of Villanova, Montpellier's most distinguished professor, mentioned Hector the Englishman as the author of a recipe in his *Breviarium*.[118] Henry of Winchester was a medical master at Montpellier in the early thirteenth century and was probably the author of a Latin phlebotomy text that was translated into Middle English.[119] Numerous thirteenth-century apothecaries seem to have come from Montpellier, although not necessarily from the university.[120] Most notable was Peter of Montpellier, a royal apothecary, who treated the redoubtable Italian physician Pancio da Controne at Hoxne Manor in Suffolk in 1329.[121]

The University of Paris apparently drew the majority of English medical men who studied abroad. The diplomat, physician, mathematician, and cardinal Hugh of Evesham probably studied at Paris in the mid-thirteenth century, as did John of Cella late in the twelfth century.[122] Paris seems to have been a popular destination for medical students in the fifteenth century. John Kim studied medicine first at Cambridge and then at Paris in the second quarter of the fifteenth century, with the help of royal and noble patrons.[123] The first transfer student in medicine from Oxford may have been Stephen of Cornwall, who first studied arts at Oxford in the early fourteenth century and left for Paris to obtain his medical doctorate.[124] Thomas Broun attempted and failed to transfer credit for his medical study from Oxford to Paris in 1396.[125]

The other great magnet for foreign travel, and a generator of documentary records, was the military campaign. In a letter written by Martin de Pateshull, chief justice of the court of Common Pleas, a physician named Master Thomas is recommended to attend the royal army because "in the siege of castles, medics are necessary, and especially ones who know how to cure wounds."[126] Royal and noble persons were usually accompanied on foreign campaigns by physicians and surgeons. As is the case with foreign medical education, the intellectual impact of foreign medical experience on English practitioners is difficult to assess; however, foreign travel must have served to integrate English practitioners into a larger world of experience, experience they brought back to their native country.

The Crusades, most of which took place from the eleventh through the thirteenth centuries, were military expeditions as well as religious pilgrimages. It is difficult to trace the movements of individual medical practitioners with their military patrons along the route to Jerusalem. Even so, military religious orders like the Knights Hospitallers seem to have trained medical practitioners in England to treat the ill and wounded of their own group.[127]

Richard I was in all likelihood accompanied on the Third Crusade by the aforementioned Master Malger, *medicus*, who later became bishop of Worcester in about 1200. Malger lived in England but probably was French.[128] Thomas, a monk of St. Albans, accompanied the earl of Arundel to the Holy Land as his physician and, on his death there, had the earl's body preserved and returned to England for burial. He died in 1248, after being made prior of Wymondham, near Norwich, where he had arranged for his patron's burial.[129] The cleric Master John de Brideport, physician to William de Valence, earl of Pembroke, seems to have accompanied his master to the Holy Land along with Edward I in 1270. He received a lifetime appointment as parson of Axeminster in 1277.[130] In 1392 a certain John, serving the future Henry IV as his physician, was paid for drugs in Gdánsk while accompanying his master on a crusade through Prussia.[131]

One might hope for evidence of the development of surgical expertise during the heat of foreign battles, but no testimony survives that this took place. John Bradmore did indeed develop a surgical instrument for the removal of an arrow from the head of the future Henry V in 1403, but that happened at the battle of Shrewsbury, which is in England.[132] Instead, the evidence that remains of surgical practice shows that royal and noble persons were usually accompanied by surgeons on foreign campaigns, which sometimes involved combat. What these surgeons actually did more often than not can only be conjectured. The generous remuneration they gained for this service, however, is beyond dispute.

Henry III took Thomas de Weseham with him to Gascony about 1253, and showered him and his wife, Cristiana, with gifts and privileges throughout his life, one of which may have included a knighthood for Thomas. Henry gained for him the right to mint silver pennies and settled his debts with Jewish moneylenders.[133] Master Martin, *surgicus*, was paid more than £13 in about 1341 at the behest of Edward III for his service overseas, although exactly where is not recorded.[134]

The renewal of the campaigns of the Hundred Years' War in 1415 gave rise to the best-documented medical expedition from England to the Continent yet studied. The London surgeon Thomas Morstede contracted with Henry V in 1415 to accompany him to France with twelve surgeons and three archers, along with a cart and horses carrying medical supplies.[135] The physician and cleric Nicholas Colnet, fellow of Merton College, Oxford, contracted with Henry under similar terms.[136] A year later, Morstede again accompanied the king to France, this time with craftsmen to make and repair surgical instruments. On his return to England, Morstede gained numerous royal preferments and married. According to one historian, he was among the wealthiest men of his time.[137]

Finally, it would appear that some English medical practitioners went abroad never to return. About 1250 an English surgeon, Peter Arderne, was recorded practicing in Paris. It is not known whether he was related to the famous English surgeon John of Arderne.[138] There is also mention of William the Englishman, citizen of Marseilles, who was a physician, astrologer, and prolific author.[139] William Valponi, of English origin, was physician to the dowager countess of Savoy, was married, and was executed for counterfeiting coin in 1391.[140]

CONCLUSION

Britain is an island, but links of commerce and the church tied it to the European continent in ways that shaped how medicine was understood. As was the case with native English people, foreign healers more often than not practiced medicine only part-time: they were churchmen and doctors, moneylenders and doctors, wool traders and doctors. Most foreign practitioners (including Jews) were in some sense entrepreneurs, whose marketable skills included the practice of learned medicine. The shift from a feudal economy that involved ties of obligation between a lord and his man to a market economy that involved buying and selling of goods and services acted to open opportunities for these foreign practitioners.

If the status of foreign practitioners is viewed from another aspect, it seems clear that patrons of medicine preferred treatment from foreigners coming from countries that could boast a medical university. This is especially clear in the later medieval period. Italian, French, and Iberian practitioners appear frequently, whereas Germans, although without a doubt present in large numbers by reason of their links with trade, are all but absent from the records of foreign medical practice. Finally, patrons of foreign medical practitioners were often foreigners themselves, preferring doctors from their native lands. English nobles often took foreign brides or, like Richard I, spent little time in England.

Learned practitioners were almost all clerics until the later fifteenth century, and their clerical status allowed them to move relatively freely to the European continent for education under the patronage of the church. Foreign study was especially important for physicians because medical faculties at Oxford and Cambridge remained small as compared to those at Paris, Bologna, Montpellier, and Padua. Indeed, the dominance of non-English medical faculties assured that the English ones remained insignificant through the end of the fifteenth century.

CHAPTER III

The Medieval English Medical Text

MEDICAL TEXTS from the English Middle Ages survive in large numbers and are the most obvious source of knowledge about the medicine of the period. These documents come in many forms and languages, from the gigantic Latin *Compendium medicine* (Compendium of medicine) of Gilbert Eagle (Gilbertus Anglicus) to short recipes and charms written in vernacular languages like English or French. Long texts often stood alone, but the shorter ones could be bound together with other medical texts or with material that, from a modern perspective, had little, if anything, to do with healing.

Medical texts in English, either in Old English (also called Anglo-Saxon), the common language before the Norman Conquest, or in Middle English, written and spoken from the twelfth through the fifteenth centuries, have been relatively well studied.[1] Philologists have also turned their attention to medical texts in Anglo-Norman, the language written and spoken by the conquering nobility from France.[2] Anglo-Latin medical texts, which were for the most part the province of educated men of clerical training, have been studied less, but they provide important testament to the state of medieval English medical learning.

Medical learning that was written down is bound closely with levels of education: one assumes that the existence of a text at least implied the existence of someone who could read it, or read it to other people. Given the assumption of a reading public, the audience for text-based medicine must have been relatively small; however, the frequent shifts of language encountered in these texts suggest a varied and eager readership.

The survival of medical texts in Latin and medical texts in various English vernaculars might seem to imply that the former represented the record of educated, theory-based medicine, while the latter represented the record of folk practice. This is not the case. The two traditions—Latin and vernacular—are closely interrelated. Although learned, university-style medicine was always written in Latin, medical texts in the vernacular were almost always translations of Latin originals.[3] So-called folk practice—the use of remedies derived from experience alone—can be found in both Latin and vernacular, as can charms and prayers.

The very fact that medical knowledge was written down makes it a part of learned tradition, whether in Latin or in the vernacular. In this sense, at

least, all medical texts must be considered together as a part of elite intellectual culture. It is also a well-founded truism of medieval English culture
that texts, creative though they may have been in form and content, were
never entirely "original": every piece owed a distinctive debt to other written sources. This is especially true for medieval English medical writings,
since compilation and translation from other sources were the principal
methods of textual production.[4]

Medieval English medical texts do not lend themselves to classification
by language: texts in Latin could be charms and prayers, whereas vernacular ones could be translations of learned, university-style writings. One distinction, albeit a sometimes fuzzy one, does emerge from a survey of the
written records of medieval English medicine. In general, texts can be divided into those that derive ultimately from ancient Greek sources, translated and adapted by Islamic scholars into Arabic and then into scholastic
Latin for use in universities; and Roman or humanistic, those derived from
the writings of educated patriarchs like Pliny or the Elder Cato, which re-
lied on simple remedies, charms, and traditional wisdom. The latter—aristocratic and familial medicine often found in encyclopedic form with other
types of useful knowledge—met the relatively simple needs of monastic
communities. Aristocratic, encyclopedic medicine enjoyed an unbroken
tradition in England from the time of the Anglo-Saxons, lasted beyond the
end of the medieval period, and seemed to some educated medical writers
to be the medicine not only of the ancient Roman paterfamilias but of the
Old Testament patriarchs themselves. These two "styles" of medical writing,
the Greek/Arabic and the Roman/Anglo-Saxon or patriarchal, were never
entirely separate (Pliny, for instance, used Greek sources at times). But they
do form distinctive trends in medieval English medical writing, not just
stages in evolution toward modern medicine. As such, they serve as useful
classifications for understanding the nature of elite medical discourse.

THE ORIGINS OF GRECO-ARABIC
MEDICAL TEXTS IN LATIN

The first large body of written medicine in the West comes from the ancient
Greek city-states and is associated with the name Hippocrates. The Hippocratic corpus of texts, most of which were written between 430 and 330
B.C., helped establish medicine as a discipline that had a history, made
progress, and rested on a set of theoretical principles based on, but not
limited to, experience.[5] Ultimately what distinguished Hippocratic medicine from others was its insistence that every natural phenomenon (and
thus all diseases) had rational causes.[6] These rational causes were the subject for public debate.[7] The reasons for these causes were also subject to

refinement, because the physicians of the past knew less than the physicians of the present, and those of the present less than those of the future.[8]

Hippocratic medicine was written down, as was the philosophy of the ancient Greeks. This very fact gave Hippocratic medicine an enormous advantage over competing types of healing that did not leave much written record, for instance, healing by resorting to the help of the gods.[9] Indeed, it was obvious from their writings that Hippocratic physicians considered various kinds of religious and mystical practitioners to be their competitors. This is not to say that Hippocratic physicians were irreligious. On the contrary, they were at pains to demonstrate their own piety and the impiety of their competitors.[10] What in the end distinguished Hippocratic physicians from their rivals was that their writings survived, like those of Plato, Aristotle, and their commentators.[11]

The most distinguished reader of the Hippocratic corpus of texts was another Greek, the physician Galen, who served as philosopher to the Stoic Roman emperor Marcus Aurelius. Galen extolled Hippocrates as a great physician, almost a god, but having conceded that, was anxious to demonstrate how he himself knew more.[12] Galen was probably the most prolific writer of antiquity, covering the whole of rational medicine, from surgery to anatomy to pharmacy. He, like the Hippocratic physicians, demonstrated his medical knowledge publicly, and argued at length that he was not only Hippocrates' successor but Aristotle's as well.[13]

Galen insisted, against those who would relegate the physician to a lowly status with other craftsmen, that the best doctor was also a philosopher and, more than that, a philanthropist, who dispensed his medical knowledge to his familiars for the love of humanity alone and without regard for payment. Assumed in Galen's sort of medicine was a Stoic detachment from the hurly-burly of the marketplace. Galen's physician was a wealthy gentleman of great learning, freed by his wealth from the exigencies of making a living or rearing a family.[14]

Galen wrote in Greek, which even under the Roman Empire remained the language of philosophical learning. After the disintegration and division of the empire, the ability to read Greek was almost lost in the West, even though the Eastern Empire, Byzantium, carried on that tradition. But political and religious differences acted to isolate the Eastern and Western Empires. The copying of Greek medical texts continued under Byzantium, but the Western Empire for the most part was unable to appreciate this work in its original language.[15]

The military and religious triumphs of the prophet Muhammad transformed the culture of much of the Mediterranean world. Islamic rulers funded vast educational enterprises, including schools of translation, where the philosophical and medical texts of the Greeks were examined, translated, and adapted to Islamic culture. Islamic scholars made compilations of Greek philosophical medicine, with commentaries they prepared themselves, written in Arabic.[16] The most famous of these compendiums was the *Canon* of the Persian philosopher Ibn Sina (Avicenna), a huge text so learned and well organized that it dominated scholarly medicine well into the Renaissance.[17]

Western scholars, usually from the Iberian Peninsula or Italy, began to collect and translate Arabic medical texts in the twelfth century as part of a general enterprise in Western Christendom to recover and examine the philosophical learning of the ancient Greeks, especially Aristotle.[18] Among the first centers of philosophic medical learning in the West was Salerno, in southern Italy, near the famous Benedictine monastery of Monte Cassino. At the end of the eleventh century, Constantine the African assembled a school of translators who helped bring philosophical medicine back into the Latin-speaking world. These writings in Latin formed the basis of the curriculum of the so-called School of Salerno, the first medical university in the West.[19]

What Constantine and those like him brought to the West was not a mere reconstruction of Greek learning; rather, it was the product of Islamic understanding of the ancient Greeks. Islamic philosophers systematized Greek medical learning to make it easier to teach (most obviously by translating this learning into Arabic). They also added their own observations about astrology and alchemy, advancing Western knowledge of these and other subjects far beyond what it had been in Galen's time.[20] Western medicine from the twelfth century onward, then, was part of a more widespread interest in the culture of Islam: its philosophy, its art, its poetry, and its technical knowledge. Western armies may have repulsed the armies of Islam, but Western scholars later eagerly embraced the impressive learning of the very people they had fought so hard to defeat.

ARABIC MEDICAL LEARNING IN ENGLAND

From the end of the eleventh century, Western scholars and travelers were able to take increasing interest in the culture of Islam. The best-known contact was through the Crusades, which were ostensibly an attempt by Western Christians to win the Holy Land back from the Saracens. Romantic poetry flourished from the twelfth century onward, especially in France, as tales of Christian knights fighting offending Muslims became a staple of elite society. So-called courtly love, the elaborate ritual of approach and rebuke between a lady and gentleman, also became a well-documented phenomenon in cultured northern European society. Many scholars have suggested Islamic models for these poems and the courtly behavior that they suggest.[21] The Crusades are best understood as campaigns of warfare and looting, not of cultural exchange. More important to learned medicine were English scholars' contacts with Spain and Sicily, where Arabic, Jewish, Greek, and Western Christian learning flourished in an atmosphere of relative toleration.[22] Especially important for the dissemination of Arabic scientific learning to the West was the Christian reconquest of the Spanish city of Toledo, a great center of translation, in 1085.[23]

Scientific learning, of which learned medicine was a part, likewise was transformed by the West's discovery of Islamic scholarship. In England, scholars like Adelard of Bath, Alfred of Sareshel, John Blund, and the Jewish convert Petrus Alponsi brought learning about the natural sciences from the European continent largely by means of translations from Arabic.[24] For these men medicine was not a subject to be taught in a separate medical faculty the way it was at the great Italian and French universities of the time. Instead, their interest in medicine grew out of study of Aristotle's natural sciences, which were typically taught at the undergraduate level as part of a study of philosophy.[25] For example, Alfred of Sareshel (fl. 1200) wrote a learned Latin commentary on the motion of the heart dedicated to Alexander Neckam sometime before 1217.[26] Although he showed some familiarity with medical writers, citing Galen, Hippocrates, Isaac, and Johannitius in a way that indicated familiarity with the Salernitan medical curriculum sometimes called *articella*, his best authorities were Aristotle and his natural philosophical texts.[27]

A significant break with the undergraduate philosophical tradition of medical learning in England came with the assembly of the *Compendium medicine* by Gilbertus Anglicus, England's first major medical writer. The *Compendium*, written about 1230, attempted to cover all of medicine, and cited numerous Arabic medical authorities, especially Avicenna and Averroes.[28] Gilbert himself was almost certainly a priest, and is cited at least once as royal physician to King John. The earliest manuscript of his book, dated 1271, names him Gilbertus de Aquila, Anglicus (Gilbert Eagle, Englishman), and this has been accepted as an indication he was a member of a prominent Anglo-Norman family by that name.[29]

As the first major representative of medical Arabism in England, it would be helpful to know where Gilbert had studied. Scholars have made numerous suggestions, including Paris and Salerno, but evidence is inconclusive. He need not have studied medicine at a university at all. Agostino Paravicini Bagliani has documented a flourishing intellectual community at the papal court that included English physicians and philosophers,[30] and Gilbert may have been one of them. Certainly he was in Rome in 1214.[31] Gilbert mentioned with admiration the equally problematic medical writer Richardus Anglicus, calling him "of all the doctors the most learned and experienced" [omnium doctorum doctissimus et expertissimus].[32] No other of Gilbert's medical writers was praised by him so warmly. Richard was said by one contemporary to have been a papal physician, as well as a doctor at the medical university town of Montpellier in the south of France.[33] The knotty problem of where Gilbert learned his medicine still lacks a definitive answer, and perhaps our notions about where advanced medical learning took place will have to be examined again.

Gilbert's book is divided into seven chapters, beginning with one on fevers, because fevers affect the body as a whole. Detailed and packed with learned commentary, the treatise seems to imply that fever is an affliction of the soul, in the Aristotelian philosophical and not the Christian religious sense. His principal authority is Avicenna. Other chapters on various parts of the body follow, from the head downward. Gilbert intended to include all medical knowledge available to him, arranged for easy reference, including learned theory and ranging to recipes, charms, and prayers. The poet Geoffrey Chaucer, writing near the end of the fourteenth century, included Gilbert as the first of three authoritative writers of medical compendia, the other two being Bernard Gordon, the famous Montpellier professor, and John of Gaddesden, who flourished in England a century after Gilbert's time.[34]

Gilbert's compendium does not differ greatly from other medical collections of the later Middle Ages, including those of Gaddesden and Bernard mentioned above. After the chapter on fevers, each body part is treated from head downward, with rules for diagnosis and recipes for treatment given for each. For instance, in the case of worms in the ears, "Sometimes worms crop up in the ears, especially ears that are pus-filled or ulcerated, . . . or sometimes a worm or some other creeping thing enters into the ear."[35] "Ringing in the ears," Gilbert continued, "comes from windiness enclosed in hollows of the ears that has no way out because of its thickness."[36] Various authorities are weighed and remedies offered, based for the most part on herbal preparations taken from learned scholastic sources.[37]

Gilbert also dealt with matters that may seem to modern sensibilities outside the scope of a medical text, but were in fact typical of many medieval medical compendiums. For instance, Gilbert's compendium devoted quite a bit of space to the arrangement and beautification of women's hair, because, Gilbert noted, "women are anxious to please men" [mulieres viris placere student].[38] Passages like these hint strongly at a female readership, or at least a readership of men eager to please their female patrons. Male vanity was not neglected either. A few paragraphs along, the doctor offered advice to men on how to make their beards grow thick.[39] The devotion of a scholastic physician to the adornment of his patrons may strike some as odd; however, Gilbert himself noted in his introductory material to his chapter on fevers that the *medicus* acted as a "minister of nature" [minister nature].[40]

Not all of Gilbert's sources were scholastic. The French surgeon Guy de Chauliac remarked archly in 1363 that he did not bother to present unlearned remedies and charms, because plenty could be found in Gilbert's work.[41] Gilbert indeed did not scruple to draw from whatever healing sources with which he was familiar. Prayers and charms were not as abundant as Guy perhaps wanted to imply, but they are suggested both as a first resort and when other measures failed.

For instance, in his chapter on wounds, Gilbert recommended the usual remedies of ointments, oils, and other unremarkable treatments. Then, he noted that some people believe that all wounds (*plagas*) could be cured just by a divine charm (*diuino carmine*).[42] Gilbert subsequently recited the story of three brothers who were going along the road, when Jesus met them and asked them where they were going. One said that they were on their way to the Mount of Olives, collecting herbs for blows and wounds. Jesus invited them to follow him and to believe in him through the crucifixion and through the milk of the virgin mother (*per lac mulieris virginis*). He further advised them to take wool cut from a sheep (*accipite lanam succidam ouis*) and olive oil and to place it on wounds. A comparison was made between the wound in Christ's side and the wound under treatment. Just as Jesus' wound "did not long bleed, nor did it erode, nor hurt, nor fester, let not this wound do so" [nec diu sanguinauit nec rodanauit nec doluit nec putredinem fecit nec faciat plaga ista]. The Pater Noster was to be said three times.[43] Gilbert also drew upon biblical sources whenever possible. Gilbert's cure for weak eyesight, for instance, is reminiscent of the ritual sacrifice of a bird in an earthenware bowl used to cleanse a house of skin disease or mold.[44]

Gilbert's claims for his own medical experience and on sensory data were frequent and strenuous. In his introductory material, he wrote of the doctor "following the judgment of sense" [sequens iudicium sensus].[45] Later on, he referred to his own repeated experience (*experientia mihi sepius confirmauit*) in the use of "imperial purge" [kataricum imperiale].[46] Gilbert's devotion to experience was affirmed in another of his medical writings, a commentary on the uroscopy of Giles of Corbeil. In the commentary, Gilbert affirmed that the faculty of uroscopy could "not be demonstrated by language."[47]

Charles Talbot has compared the *Compendium* to the *Summa theologica* of Gilbert's younger contemporary Thomas Aquinas, and the comparison seems apt.[48] Gilbert's book, save for the first chapter on fevers, is not that of a university professor like Taddeo Alderotti. Gilbert sought out the best texts of his time, but did not try to criticize or analyze them in any depth. Like the English medical writers who followed after him—John of Gaddesden and Simon Bredon—Gilbert saw the need for assembly and arrangement more than analysis and criticism. He collected more medical recipes than any writer of the English Middle Ages before the fifteenth century, and his recipes, not his work on fevers, gave him lasting fame. The Italian surgeon Theodoric of Lucca cited a recipe of his in about 1267,[49] and the recipes in his six latter chapters were translated into English perhaps at the end of the fourteenth century.[50] University professors owned his book, and cited it in their work,[51] but Gilbert himself never seems to have taught at any university.

Medical study at the two English universities of Oxford and Cambridge did not really begin as a separate discipline in its own faculty until fifty years after Gilbert's death. At that time, medicine became established as a graduate faculty, along with theology and canon and civil law, to be studied after a thorough grounding in the undergraduate liberal arts. England's medical faculties were never large or very important, as compared to that at the University of Paris, on which English universities were modeled. Foreign physicians seem to have dominated elite practice, and it is thus not surprising that the first few medical texts to emerge from these faculties were attempts to adapt Continental medical learning to an English audience.

English universities' first and only major medical writer was John of Gaddesden, whose *Rosa medicinae* (Rose of medicine) was written somewhere around 1320. Gaddesden was a Merton College, Oxford–educated physician with royal and noble patrons. His book is a compendium; that is, it was written to bring together medical knowledge from a number of different sources in an easily understandable format.[52] Gaddesden wrote his book in Latin, and directed it explicitly to surgeons and physicians, both poor and rich.[53] This is in itself interesting. Surgery was not taught formally at Oxford or Cambridge, and this suggests that Gaddesden was addressing an audience in Latin outside the formal teaching of the university.

Gaddesden began his compendium with the admonition, taken from Galen, that one ought not enter into the halls of princes without a knowledge of books. Continuing to cite Galen, Gaddesden further advised that the physician could come close to God through learning.[54] What followed was a discussion of learned medicine based not on Aristotle the philosopher, as were Blund's and Alfred's works, but on Galen the physician, perhaps reflecting a deliberate departure from medicine as part of the arts curriculum to medicine as its own graduate faculty. Gaddesden began with a study of fevers. He then moved to a study of the various organ systems, beginning with the brain and covering the eyes, ears, nose, mouth and tongue, heart, stomach, liver, kidneys, intestines, womb, reproduction in women, male organs, joints, abscesses and swellings, dislocations, nerves, skin diseases, poisons, advice for travelers, and the compounding of medicines.

Gaddesden, like most scholastic thinkers, was careful to shape his medical diagnoses and treatments to the individual characteristics of each patient. The falling sickness (epilepsy) has a different prognosis for pregnant women and children,[55] whereas trembling of the heart (*cardica passio*) often affected young people.[56] Sterility has two results: men do not generate and women do not conceive.[57] A regimen of health is important in stomach diseases, and one ought to vary the quantity of food and wine intaken according to age, as was advised by Aristotle in his letter to Alexander the Great (i.e., the *Secretum secretorum*) and according to Avicenna's regimen of health.[58] His advice to travelers applied to people who went to war, on pilgrimages, to fairs, to see friends, or to visit the sick the way doctors did ("sicut medici faciunt").[59]

It would be difficult to credit Gaddesden with much originality: one historian noted fifteen hundred citations to more than forty authors, about five hundred of those to Avicenna and slightly fewer to Galen. Most of the rest are to writers educated at Montpellier and Paris.[60] But the text does show particular English characteristics. For instance, Gaddesden noted that certain kinds of pustules (*variole*) "they call in English 'measles' " [vocant anglice mesles].[61]

Another notable English medical Arabist was the surgeon John of Arderne. Unlike Gaddesden, Arderne was not a professor; indeed, there is no evidence he ever attended university at all. Arderne wrote a *Practica* in Latin sometime in the 1370s that by and large concerned his adaptation of the operation for anal fistula ultimately derived from Arabic sources.[62] Both Gaddesden and Arderne were associated with the great military campaigner Edward the Black Prince, and it is possible these medical practitioners were charged with creating an English tradition of practical medical texts.[63] Arderne was especially successful in reaching a wide audience of readers. His surgery was translated into English several times not long after it was written; some of these translations contain illustrations of Arderne's operation and its instruments—some of the most unusual surviving testaments to the nature of medieval surgery.[64] Equally remarkable are the numerous patients Arderne named. Many can be identified exactly, and among them are several members of the nobility.[65] If Arderne's word is to be believed, Arabic surgical methods were put into practice in medieval England among elite patrons.

Besides Gaddesden, the university professor and medical generalist, and Arderne, the layman and surgical specialist, was Mertonian Simon Bredon, M.D., who wrote on uroscopy, pharmacy, and the pulse. Simon Bredon is best known for his work in the Oxford arts faculty as a mathematician and astronomer. His only medical work, the *Trifolium*, survives in a single incom-

plete manuscript, which dates from the fifteenth century.[66] Its date of composition is unknown (Bredon died in 1372). The text ends abruptly in the
section on pulses at the end of a folio. This may indicate that Digby 160 is
an incomplete exemplar of a finished work that does not survive in its en-
tirety. The section on urines is by far the longest, covering folios 102–172v.[67]
The section on medicines and complexions runs from folio 173 to 219,
and the section on pulses ends at the bottom of folio 222v.[68]

Bredon, like Gaddesden, was a cleric and seems to have intended his
work as a compendium of citations from the best authorities composed for
his fellow scholars. Unlike Gaddesden, however, Bredon dealt only with
the traditional interests of the physician and not with surgery. Also unlike
Gaddesden, Bredon adopted the mathematically based Aristotelian medicine popular at the time in France, especially at the University of Montpellier.[69] Bredon planned his book as a threefold regimen,[70] giving advice on
uroscopy, pharmacy, and the pulse, the last of which was believed to indicate the state of the body's innate heat, the basis of life. His plan was apparently taken from that of the French courtly physician Giles of Corbeil, who
wrote on the same subjects a century before.

Bredon's work is interesting, although not for its originality: the *Trifolium*
is little more than a series of citations in Latin from Greek and Arabic
sources. Page after page is covered with lists of drugs and their qualities, as
well as learned citations. A long section on prognosis from urines, covering
folios 112v–147v, contains a series of short predictions taken for the most
part from Isaac Israeli. Other sources include the *Pantegni*, Theophilus,
Gilbertus Anglicus, Giles of Corbeil, Walter Agilon, Bernard Gordon, and
Galen on prognosis.

Bredon's text shows how learned medicine was not autonomous but instead was intimately connected with other disciplines. Bredon's pharmacy
is mathematized, adopting a complex system of "degrees" of heat and cold-
ness for every drug. His uroscopy, like his astrology, was prognostic, divin-
ing the nature of the physical universe by hidden signs only the trained eye
could detect. For Bredon, as for so many of the best university-educated
physicians on the European continent, mathematics, not the recipe-based
arrangements of diseases and cures offered by physicians like Gaddesden,
was the best medicine.

Bredon's *Trifolium*, unfinished, short, and often cryptic, represented the
best English medicine had to rival the high state of medical learning demonstrated at Montpellier or Bologna. Whereas the close association of the
arts and medical faculties at those two universities seems to have favored
and strengthened medicine, in England the association seems to have ben-
efited the arts. Bredon's principal textual legacy was to the liberal arts,
especially mathematics and astronomy/astrology, not to medicine.

THE ORIGINS OF THE ENCYCLOPEDIC
MEDICAL TRADITION IN ENGLAND

Gaddesden and Bredon were both university-educated medical doctors and, like Arderne, the learned surgeon, or Gilbert, the learned cleric, approached medicine from some degree of specialization. All four were known to have served as medical practitioners to elite patrons, and all were writing for other healers. Many important English medical writers wrote about learned medicine from another perspective: as a part of general knowledge. In incorporating medical learning with other types of learning, these writers were following an ancient tradition that extended back before the rise of universities in the twelfth century and carried on beyond it.

The encyclopedic tradition was known to medieval English people through ancient Roman examples. Patricians like the elder Cato and Pliny the Elder wrote about medicine as part of the sort of knowledge the paterfamilias ought to have. For them, simple remedies were part of traditional learning about estate management. These writers were aware of the accomplishments of Greek philosophical physicians, but found their concern with the body excessive, even effeminate. In Pliny's encyclopedia *Historia naturalis* (Natural history), the writer denounced the repellent foreign ways of Greek medicine and their malign effects on once great Rome: "It is certainly true that our degeneracy, due to medicine more than to anything else, proves daily that Cato was a genuine prophet and oracle when he stated that it is enough to dip into the works of Greek brains without making a close study of them."[71] Pliny's own remedies were, above all, things based on nature lore and Roman tradition. We would call them folk medicine, magic, or old wives' tales,[72] and yet they are some of the most respected records of written medicine that survive in western Europe.[73]

The disregard Romans like Cato and Pliny had for what they felt to be excessive bodily concerns, the respect for family life, and the reverence they held for the aged man were the antithesis of Greek idealization of the young male athlete, an obsession Pliny was clear would lead to degeneracy of the worst sort. Indeed, it is remarkable that, while Greek thinkers included gymnastics among the liberal arts—the activities proper to a gentleman—the Romans typically left gymnastics out.[74]

During the social and cultural disorganization that accompanied the decline of Roman authority in the West, much of the Roman encyclopedic tradition perished. Celsus and Varro, who included a large amount of medical material in their encyclopedias, were lost.[75] But the works of writers like Pliny, Latin compilations of late antiquity, and a host of anonymous texts attributed to various ancients survived, especially in monastic communities.[76] Most notable of these monastic retreats was one on the Benedictine

model at Vivarium near Rome, where the senator Cassiodorus, who flourished under the barbarian emperor Theodoric, retired from public life in
540. Cassiodorus ordered his monks to learn about medicinal herbs, and
he had medical texts copied, including works attributed (perhaps wrongly)
to Galen, Hippocrates, the pharmacist Dioscorides, and Caelius.[77]

The medicine of the Roman paterfamilias, with its simple remedies and
charms, Stoic retirement, communal living under a male leader, and disin-
terest in material wealth, transferred well to a Christian context, although
the pagan charms were replaced by Christian ones.[78] Roman or monastic
medicine did not reflect a complex vision of the role of humans in nature
the way Greek philosophical medicine did. Rather, it was remedy-oriented:
simple recipes for simple diseases, incorporating charms and prayers,
which reflected a very ancient medical tradition.[79] For example, the Benedictine rule, written shortly before Cassiodorus's retirement, recommended only special food and isolation for the ill, in the charge of the
abbot and his second-in-command, the cellarer. This care was as much for
the spiritual benefit of the caregiver as it was for the ill man.[80]

THE ENCYCLOPEDIC TRADITION IN ENGLAND

The earliest evidence of medical texts, or texts containing some medical
material, comes from Anglo-Saxon England. Medical knowledge, like
Christianity and the Latin language, had to be brought in across the English Channel, and the Anglo-Saxons represent one of many "importa-
tions" of medical knowledge from the European continent. The Anglo-
Saxons arrived beginning probably in the fifth century of the common era,
and displaced the Britons, whose descendants remain in Scotland, Ireland,
Wales, and Brittany. The language of the Anglo-Saxons, which consisted of
several dialects, is called Old English. The educated clergy also spoke and
wrote Latin. One of the earliest medieval encyclopedias was that of the
Venerable Bede, who wrote his *De natura rerum* (On the nature of things)
in the opening years of the eighth century, based on Pliny and Isidore
of Seville. It was created as a teaching text, presenting knowledge of the
natural world as part of an exegesis of the Hexaemeron (six days of Creation).[81] Modern readers are most familiar with the Old English of the poetic adventure *Beowulf* and similar poems, but many other types of writings
remain in Old English too. Medical material survives in several manuscripts, and the corpus of Old English texts contains some of the earliest
surviving medical material in a Western vernacular language. Medical texts
in Old English, for the most part recipes, charms, and prayers, existed side
by side in manuscripts.[82]

The copying of manuscripts in Anglo-Saxon England was in essence a monastic activity, and medicine was part of a Christian mission. Not surprisingly, these Anglo-Saxon Christians took as their example the monastic copyists of Europe: they reproduced a wide range of texts, among them medical writings. The patient work of Old English philologists has demonstrated beyond doubt the debt Anglo-Saxon medical manuscripts (copied in England between the late eighth and late eleventh centuries) owed to European models.[83] These Anglo-Saxon Christians were the intellectual children not only of the Roman Catholic Church but of the decayed Latin-speaking Roman Empire, and their choice of texts mirrors an intellectual loyalty to their Roman origins. Anglo-Saxon medical manuscripts very much reflect the traditional charms and recipes typified by Pliny and by similar texts attributed to him. What has not usually been appreciated, however, is the willingness Anglo-Saxon copyists showed, after the Roman paterfamilias, to copy down traditional native cures and to incorporate them into collections assembled from continental European sources.[84] Anglo-Saxon medical manuscripts thus look very much like medical encyclopedias, assembled from bits and pieces of lore known to various copyists as well as pieces of texts jotted down from other manuscripts.[85]

Medical material from Anglo-Saxon England survives in monastic encyclopedias and chronicles, in the lives of famous persons, both of which were written in Latin,[86] and in medical manuscripts in Latin and Old English.[87] All these sources contain religious and magical healing, both pagan and Christian,[88] and others are witness to material on gynecology, the growth of the child,[89] and surgery.[90] The most commonly found type of medical material is the herbal recipe.[91]

The most intensively studied witness to learned medicine in Anglo-Saxon England is the so-called Leechbook of Bald, which occupies the first 108 folios of London, British Library, Royal MS 12.D.XVII, copied probably at Winchester, the famous center of monastic learning, about 950.[92] The work gets its name from a metrical colophon on folio 109 stating that a certain Bald had it compiled.[93] The work is probably a duplicate of one composed at the court of King Alfred, a great patron of translation from Latin into Old English, at the end of the ninth century.[94] The remainder of Royal MS 12.D.XVII is occupied by another medical collection copied by the same scribe and known to scholars as Leechbook III. It is a medical miscellany, much less well-organized than the Leechbook of Bald, and founded on a different set of sources.[95]

The Leechbook has two parts that are well integrated textually, the first a list of diseases and remedies arranged in the familiar format of "top-to-toe," the second a list of remedies for diseases of the digestive system.[96] Some of the remedies are untranslated Old Irish, probably indicating an importation by English students who returned after study in that celebrated center of learning.[97] The primary language of the Leechbook is Old English. Most of the remedies are herbal, and of Mediterranean origin.[98] Some charms, native or from learned sources, were also incorporated.[99] Adams and Deegan have demonstrated that the principal source for the Leechbook is ultimately Pliny's *Historia naturalis*, which came to the Old English translator through a number of intermediary Latin epitomes. Other sources are late antique writers like Marcellus and the Latin translation of Alexander of Tralles.[100] At some point, these Latin sources were translated into Old English, as was so much of Christian learning from across the channel.[101]

MEDICINE AND THE ENCYCLOPEDIC TRADITION
AFTER THE NORMAN CONQUEST

When the bodies of Anglo-Saxon learning—Latin and Old English—are considered together, they reflect an attempt at encyclopedic coverage, a summary of all useful knowledge. A full-blown encyclopedic tradition, however, was not transplanted to England until after the Norman Conquest, when the first comprehensive encyclopedias were produced by scholars associated with the young continental European universities. As was true with the ancient encyclopedists, such as Pliny, Varro, and Celsus, medicine was always included in English encyclopedias as a part of general knowledge.

St. Isidore (d. 636), the encyclopedic writer and bishop of Seville, asserted in his encyclopedia *Etymologies* (4.13) that medicine embraced all other subjects, including grammar, rhetoric, dialectic, arithmetic, geometry, music, and astrology—the disciplines that became the mainstays of the undergraduate arts curriculum.[102] Isidore also remarked in the same passage that medicine was a "second philosophy," an advancement on the natural philosophy that would later be a part of that undergraduate curriculum. Isidore was in all likelihood alluding to Aristotle's famous remark in the *Liber de sensu*: where natural philosophy ends, there medicine begins, and natural philosophy must supply the first principles of health and disease.[103] This if nothing else assured that the subject would not be neglected by subsequent Christian writers.

Alexander Neckam (d. 1217), a teacher and later an Austin canon, wrote an encyclopedia, *De naturis rerum*, with medical material taken from Salernitan sources.[104] Also encyclopedic in nature was the *De proprietatibus rerum* (On the properties of things) of the Franciscan Bartholomew the Englishman (Bartholomaeus Anglicus). Bartholomew imagined his long and popular encyclopedia as an aid to the study of the Bible, and it explored such diverse topics as the creation of angels, the properties of the soul, the names of plants and animals, the duties of each member of a household, and medicine.

Bartholomew's original Latin has not been well studied, but a Middle English translation of his encyclopedia, made by John Trevisa at the end of the fourteenth century, was the subject of an excellent critical edition.[105] The editors have demonstrated in a volume on Bartholomew's sources published subsequently to the edition that the author was born in England before 1200 and studied first at Oxford, then at Paris. He wrote his encyclopedia probably about 1245 while a teacher of his fellow friars at Magdeburg, in Saxony.[106]

Bartholomew's medical sources were those commonly known both at Oxford and at Paris. The most important were the translations/adaptations made by Constantine the African of writings in Arabic by tenth-century authors, including the *Pantegni* (by al-Majusi, called in Latin Haly Abbas) and the *Viaticum* (by Ibn al-Jazzar).[107] The medical material in the encyclopedia is concentrated in books 4 through 7, although other books also contain information on the human body and on medicinal substances (book 3 on the senses, books 16–18 on stones, animals, and plants, and book 19 on foods and tastes).

Constantine's work on diseases occupies book 7, and in its arrangement is typical of any number of medical texts in the School of Salerno style: from head downward.[108] Where Bartholomew departed from his medical sources and returned to the example of Isidore of Seville was in his thorough etymologies and in his use of citations from the Bible. For example, in his chapter on epilepsy, Bartholomew began by citing Mark 9:18: He fell down to the earth foaming.[109] Bartholomew continued, "The falling sickness is named epilepsy by Constantine and other authors, and this disease was called from ancient times God's wrath. As Constantine says, epilepsy [*epilepsia*] is a moist humor by which the ventricles of the brain are partially stopped; . . . This disease is called *ieranoson,* that is, the 'sacred disease,' for it affects the holy part of the body, that is, the head. And it is called *Herculeus* too, because this disease is strong as Hercules."[110]

Toward the end of the fourteenth century, England produced another Latin medical encyclopedia, the *Breviarium Bartholomei* (Abridgment of Bartholomew), by London priest John of Mirfield. The work appears to have been intended for use at the hospital of St. Bartholomew, in Smithfield, London, where John had family and clerical associations.[111] Like Gilbert Eagle's *Compendium medicine,* written more than a century before, the *Breviarium* is a work of astonishing erudition, calling on every medical authority of the day. And like the *Compendium,* the *Breviarium* incorporates a large

number of charms and prayers, especially for women's needs, a feature
that may reflect the hospital's reputation of care for unwed mothers.[112]

The details of Mirfield's life are uncertain, as was his connection with
the Austin priory of St. Bartholomew and the nearby hospital. He seems to
have been the son or close relative of a priest, William Mirfield, who was
an important attorney in the circle of Edward III and John of Gaunt.[113] In
his will, which shows him to have died early in 1407, he named his mother,
"Margaret Schadelok," as executor.[114] Hartley and Aldridge relegate the
suggestion that John was William's illegitimate son to a footnote; however,
a relationship of trust undoubtedly existed between the two men in complex land transactions involving the hospital's properties in London.[115]
What is more, some barrier seems to have prevented John's ordination to
the priesthood, which finally took place in 1395.[116] That barrier may have
been illegitimacy, and if true, John's interest in the health of unwed mothers was perhaps more than academic. He was also an associate of the famous London surgeon Adam Rous, who attended Edward III.[117] Whatever
the truth of John's life might be, he found himself under the patronage of
a powerful royal associate and in the circle of the Priory and Hospital of
St. Bartholomew, the center of a notable educational tradition, educating
local children in its own schools.[118]

As with Gilbert Eagle, there is no evidence Mirfield received a university
education, but perhaps historians have made too much of this.[119] Certainly
fourteenth-century London had another Latin medical writer, the surgeon
John Arderne, who also gained a considerable medical education without
leaving a trace of university medical study. No medical books are known to
have existed at either the priory or the hospital,[120] but a 1372 library catalog
of its collection compiled by the Austin friars at York, where the Mirfield
family originated, shows an impressive set of medical holdings, including
an *articella*; part of Avicenna's *Canon*; writings by William of Saliceto;
Averroes; Gilbert Eagle on urines; Bernard Gordon on the preservation of
human life; Taddeo Alderotti's commentary on the *Aphorisms* of Hippocrates; the *Viaticum*; *Pantegni*; Platearius; Haly Abbas; and a copy of Trotula's
work on the secrets of women.[121]

Mirfield wrote two Latin encyclopedias toward the end of this life that
reflect the dual nature of his association with the Austin priory of St. Bartholomew, a religious house, and with the hospital, which offered care to
the sick poor. The first book, *Florarium Bartholomei*, a name that implies
both an anthology and a flower garden, is a religious encyclopedia, covering the health of the spirit.[122] Mirfield devoted one chapter to the duties
of the physician, especially to deontology, or medical etiquette. Mirfield's
remarks were directed to priests like himself, who had to take care not to
injure or kill a patient during surgery or medical treatment and thus inter-

fere with their principal duties to God. Special abuse was directed against the unlettered, or those never taught by a learned man;[123] the greedy;[124] and "vile and presumptuous females" who tried to practice medicine despite their natural inability to do so.[125] Mirfield's chapter is a patchwork of citations from canon law, the Bible, and several medical authorities, especially Bernard Gordon on the preservation of human life, the pseudo-Aristotelian *Secretum secretorum*, and William of Saliceto's surgery. Most of Mirfield's medical advice concerns regimen: the regulation of diet, exercise (studied at great length), and moderate lifestyle that would promote good digestion and long life, and would certainly fit in with the monastic regimen of the priory. Not a single medicinal recipe is offered, and the chapter ends with a citation from the Book of Wisdom (Ecclesiasticus)—"For it was neither herb nor poultice that cured them, but thy all-healing word, O Lord. Thou hast the power of life and death, thou bringest a man down to the gates of death and up again" (16:12–13)—and another from Jeremiah—"Heal me, O Lord, and I shall be healed, save me and I shall be saved" (17:14).[126]

The *Florarium* presented medicine among nearly two hundred other topics, including chapters on the Holy Trinity, the sacraments, and the various Christian virtues. By contrast, Mirfield's other book, the *Breviarium Bartholomei*, devoted nearly three hundred large folios to medicine alone, in a book intended for use not at the Austin priory but at the hospital.[127]

Mirfield's purpose, like that of Gilbert Eagle and John of Gaddesden, was to construct a compendium from the most acceptable sources available to him. But unlike the other two, Mirfield was no physician. Like Pliny, he was a gatherer and arranger of texts, anxious that his reader understand that his book would present information in a form easy to consult. Greedy and ignorant physicians promised anything for money, Mirfield argued. His book would allow readers to medicate themselves, especially in the case of those diseases that were curable and not too serious.[128] His ordering of material is very much like Gilbert's or Gaddesden's: fevers, head, chest, abdomen and genitals, legs and feet. He also covered wounds and abscesses, fractures and dislocations, and the compounding of drugs, and finished with bloodletting and a regimen of health. As well as suggesting that the reader was responsible for his own household's medical treatment, Mirfield gathered other useful recipes, including one for a "powder for that warlike or diabolic instrument that commonly is termed the gun" [pulvis pro instrumento illo bellico siue diabolico quod vulgariter dicitur gunne].[129]

Mirfield's medical encyclopedia assembled a variety of sources, which he either consulted directly or cited through other sources.[130] Most of the book is indeed a summary of other authors, especially English ones like

Gaddesden, Gilbert, and Bartholomew, but on occasion the writer has introduced short recipes and anecdotes from local traditions known to him. Bishop Robert Grosseteste, the Franciscan chancellor of Oxford University, supplied a recipe for bladder stones.[131] Nicholas Tingewick (d. 1339), a priest and physician to Edward I, who had Oxford associations, was said by Mirfield to have given a widow money for her jaundice cure, consisting of crushed sheeps' lice with hydromel (honey water). He supposedly rode forty miles to visit her.[132]

The book's "Englishness" is further emphasized by the frequent reference to English words for diseases and medicines: for example, Middle English words like "sowthistil" (sowthistle),[133] "smal pokes" (glossing L. *variole*),[134] "chinca" (whooping cough in children),[135] "stiche," for a pain in the side,[136] "ryngwormes,"[137] and ulcers on the soles of the feet the vulgar call "dagges."[138] The text also contains sections entirely in Middle English, for example, one on the blood and water that come out of a wound.[139]

The sections on women and childbirth are especially detailed compared with similar medical compendia. A special recipe is offered for vomiting of pregnant women, and it is not placed in a special section on women's diseases, but in the section on the digestive system.[140] The book also makes careful distinctions between sufferers according to their gender. A man who sleeps with a woman afflicted with leprosy should wash his sexual member with his own urine.[141] Men who are sterile should say a prayer to St. Bartholomew,[142] whereas women in labor are given their own special prayers to repeat.[143]

Prayers and charms are offered without apology, mixed in with more conventional advice. Travelers are told to boil their drinking water or to distill it ("distilletur suaviter in distillatori et erit dulcis"), and also to pray to the Three Wise Men.[144] The Royal Touch is recommended as a cure for scrofula (a skin disease), and if that does not work, the sufferer is to float in a spring on the night of the Feast of St. John the Baptist.[145] Finally, prayer is recommended for things medicine was powerless to help, a practice Mirfield noted had fewer and fewer followers.[146]

Although the *Breviarium* drew on similar sources to the medical section of the *Florarium*, the two works show differing attitudes to medicine according to the audience for which they were designed. The *Florarium* was prepared for a community of friars, men who lived a well-regulated religious life. Good health lay in moderation, and the truest health was that of the spirit. The *Breviarium* was prepared for a population that was poor, secular, often transient, and sometimes women or children. People were impatient for instant cures and subject to the fraudulent practices of dishonest medical practitioners.[147] For these people, Mirfield prepared a huge encyclopedia of recipes, devoid of the moralizing and antifeminism of the *Florarium*. Learned practice, as exemplified by long citations of university

physicians, was recorded, as was what has sometimes been called folk practice—the sort of remedy Nicholas Tingewick had from the widow using the
humble louse as a cure. Prayers and charms were also incorporated, as
Mirfield sought out anything that could mitigate the suffering of the hospital's poor.

ROGER BACON AND MEDIEVAL ENGLISH REGIMENS
OF HEALTH

Ironically enough, the most powerful example of medical Arabism in medieval England was not thought to be Arabic at all: the medical sections of
the *Secretum secretorum*, reputed to be a series of letters between Aristotle
and his student Alexander the Great, but actually the work of an unknown
Islamic writer.[148] The appeal of the *Secretum* was that it offered advice to the
ultimate warrior prince on how to live well, not from an insinuating Greek
physician, but from the ultimate philosopher himself—an unchallenged
expert on ethics, clear thinking, and the nature of the physical world. The
Secretum was enormously popular in Europe, and in England was known in
Latin and in vernacular translations.

The *Secretum*, it is important to note, was not a university medical text,
or even a Christian document; instead, it offered a textual approach for
the philosophically trained to a royal or noble patron. Medical advice was
not offered in isolation. It was rather integrated into more general advice
on matters such as when to arise, what to eat, how to choose one's servants,
and the proper forms of dress and discourse.

The most celebrated exponent of the *Secretum* in England was the Franciscan Roger Bacon (d. 1294), who lauded it frequently and prepared a
commentary on the text himself.[149] In the *Secretum*, Bacon thought he saw
Aristotle the philosopher directing his aristocratic patron's regimen or
daily routine—the so-called nonnaturals: sleep and wakefulness, evacua-
tion and retention, food and drink, motion and rest, condition of the air,
and state of the emotions, the regulation of which would prolong man's
life to its natural extent.[150] Aristotle was Alexander's own countryman—not
a foreigner—acting as his moderate, moral, and educated adviser, just as
the faithful had read in Deuteronomy 17 and 18 and as John of Salisbury
had noted in his *Policraticus*.[151] If the *Secretum* did not answer the famous
question of what Athens had to do with Jerusalem, it came close. The philosopher John of Salisbury (ca. 1115–1180) wanted to demonstrate natural
justice among the writings of the patriarchs; Bacon looked there for natural
health. Scripture, the Greeks, and the Romans all seemed to point in one
direction—that godly medicine was a part of general philosophical learning, learning known to the ancients and found in books, books obscured

by the bad translations Bacon longed to redact. Just as philology could return corrupt, Babel-decayed texts to an uncorrupt state, so medicine could return man's body to its prelapsarian state before Eve yielded to the false teaching of the Father of Lies.[152] Man once knew how this restoration could be accomplished,[153] but this was forgotten and could be recovered only through the proper "decoding" of texts.[154]

Bacon's medical writings are tightly focused.[155] He confined his advice to adult men, not surprisingly, since he was a friar, and limited his medical purview to the undergraduate subjects of mathematics, astrology, philosophy, and the mechanical arts—which for him included "philosophical agriculture" (*agricultura philosophica*) and alchemy, a discipline he believed Aristotle had written of in the *Secretum*.[156] Bacon's overarching pedagogical agenda, of course, was derived from the greatest teacher of English Franciscans, Robert Grosseteste. Bacon wanted to find a place for medicine in a program of Christian education.[157]

In order to express his ideas on Christian medicine, Bacon employed a powerful metaphorical language common both to Holy Scripture and to pagan learning—redemption or renewal. Textual criticism would "redeem" corrupt texts and restore them to their original state before Babel; alchemy would return base metals to their pure state of gold; and proper medicine would restore the body to its prelapsarian state (the redemption of the fallen soul was of course another related matter). All three of these subjects—textual criticism or philology, alchemy, and medicine—are woven together in Bacon's most revealing medical works, a substantial section of the *Opus majus* and *De erroribus medicorum* (On the errors of the physicians).[158]

Exemplum 2 of the *Opus majus*, part 6, comes under the heading "scientia experimentalis," of which Bacon made medicine a part. It is the most detailed and carefully crafted of Bacon's medical writings.[159] He began by noting that some say the lengthening or shortening of life is dictated by the position of the stars, which have shifted little by little from their ideal places at the moment of Creation as the world grew older. Bacon did not know whether this was true, but he suggested instead another reason why man's life has been growing shorter (the reader is assumed to know the legendary ages of the Old Testament patriarchs), a reason suggested by the "magnificentia scientiae experimentalis" and written of covertly by Aristotle: a regimen of health. The nonnaturals are arranged in a man's temperament from infancy, and almost no physicians (*medici*) nowadays can adjust this. Fathers are corrupted and generate corrupt sons with the tendency to die young. This is not the only reason man's life is shorter than its natural extent. Sins weaken the powers of the soul, which in turn debilitate the body and hurry it along toward death. This too is passed along from father to son.[160]

The implications of what Bacon has argued here are important: the body was naturally healthy, and lack of learned attention to its regimen was the cause of physical deterioration. Nowhere did Bacon suggest that disease "attacks" the body and makes it ill. Physical deterioration was, instead, the absence of health, in the same way that Augustine had argued that evil was not an ontological entity but the absence of good: "evil is removed, not by removing any nature, or part of a nature, which had been introduced by the evil, but by healing and correcting that which had been vitiated and depraved. The will, therefore, is then truly free, when it is not the slave of vices and sins."[161] Bacon continued that men used to know what to do about premature physical deterioration: "through secret trials" [per experientias secretas] it had been discovered and written that this rapid aging is accidental (having avoidable side effects) and therefore can be treated. The medical art cannot achieve this but the experimental art can.[162]

The accidents of old age include gray hair, pallor, wrinkled skin, lots of mucus, stinking stool, sticky bleariness of the eyes, low blood and spirits, insomnia, crabbiness, absentmindedness, and a host of other unpleasant ills. Our days are numbered, as Scripture says,[163] but medical authors Dioscorides, Haly (al-Majusi), and Avicenna all say there is a medicine that will prolong life to its natural extent. They will not let on what it is, though.[164]

Bacon continued, Adam and his sons knew what to do because God told them; Aristotle hinted in the *Secretum* that God had a remedy to temper the humors, conserve health, and obviate the sufferings of old age and put it off. Saints, prophets, and patriarchs knew about this—Pliny especially—but it was hidden from common philosophers.[165] Bacon had read about this secret medicine in many places, especially in the book *De retardatione senectutis*, a work believed by many even in the medieval period to be Bacon's own.[166] He also read about it in *De regimine senum* of the Experimentator (al-Razi), who declared that the substance was born underwater and found in the viscera of long-lived animals. It was temperate in the fourth degree.[167] Whatever it was, made by alchemy (*ars alkimiae*) or by nature (Bacon noted that gold too was temperate in the fourth degree), his conviction was that the remedy would act somehow to restore the balance of the body's complexion. The remedy must have its elements mixed in perfect balance, because this will be the state of the (saints') bodies at the Resurrection—"for the equality of the elements in those bodies excludes corruption into eternity."[168]

Unlike bodies after the Resurrection, which will want nothing because their elements are perfectly in balance, Adam's body had the elements *almost* perfectly in balance. Because these elements lacked perfect balance, they strove with each other, and Adam needed nourishment.[169] In his body as a consequence of this slight imbalance was a tiny bit of corruption, and that is why he wanted the immortality that would follow if he ate the Forbidden Fruit. This fruit was deemed to have the elements almost in perfect balance, and for that reason it could carry over its "incorruption" into Adam. Sages wrote about foods or drinks that were perfectly temperate or nearly so, but the work and expense of finding out more about them by experience put people off.[170] Bacon implied, then, that Original Sin resulted as much from the promptings of Adam's stomach as of his wife.

Bacon's implications for proper, dietetic medicine are clear. Perfect health lay in a balanced complexion, which will be achieved only in the resurrected body.[171] Perfection wants nothing, but the almost perfect body, like Adam's, needs food and drink. The best food and drink Bacon wrote of in terms of its purity, simplicity, balance, and lack of corruption. It was temperate in the fourth degree—as balanced as possible.[172] Bacon offered many suggestions from his readings about what this perfecting food (or remedy) might be: gold, pearls, ambergris, rosemary flowers, something a peasant found in a jar buried in the ground, or the Forbidden Fruit. The ancients—and Pliny is the last authority named[173]—wrote of it, but more experience was needed to know for sure.

In this section from the *Opus majus*, Bacon attacked the question of proper medicine from the standpoints of natural science and Holy Scripture. His alchemical imagery of secrecy, perfection, nobility, the removal of impurities, and decoding the covert writings of ancients was combined with images of sin and resurrection to suggest that it was research into food and drink that would alleviate the accidents of old age and extend man's life to its greatest possible length.[174]

In his second major medical treatise, *De erroribus medicorum*,[175] Bacon attacked improper medicine from the standpoint of medical humanism. It is difficult to tell exactly what he used for a model in this work, but it has its closest counterpart in the first few chapters of book 29 of Pliny's *Historia naturalis*. Nearly a century after Bacon's text, the humanist poet Petrarch wrote his *Invectiva contra medicum* (Invective against physicians), at greater length but along similar lines, urging the exiled pope in Avignon to send away his many doctors and, for the sake of his health, choose only one.[176] Both the *Invectiva* and *De erroribus*, then, would seem to belong to a tradition of humanistic antiphysician invective, put forth by fierce defenders of textual scholarship.

Bacon began his bombastic diatribe in typical style, promising much but delivering considerably less. The physicians of today are guilty of thirty-six major errors and countless subsidiary ones, he began, but later decided that naming all thirty-six errors would take too long.[177] The major errors Bacon did attack fall into two related categories: errors of dependency and errors of ignorance. Good physicians should know for themselves about the quality, use, price, and efficacy of drugs. Otherwise, they are at the mercy of rustic apothecaries, "who have no intention if not to deceive them."[178] This leads to the second sort of error: ignorance—of mathematical compounding of drugs, of astrology, of alchemy, of philosophical agriculture, of natural philosophy, and especially of language, which prevents them from understanding medicine and what they ought to do.[179]

Summarizing Bacon's text is difficult, largely because it is very disorganized, wandering and doubling back on itself. But it does contain some important and revealing themes. First of all, medical writers disagree with each other all the time when they should be speaking with one voice: "Authors say the same simple medicine purges contraries, i.e. contrary humors, as when Haly says that senna purges red choler, and Avicenna in his chapter on fumitory says that it purges burnt humors, and the Latin authors say that it purges melancholy."[180] Discordance of language, then, is a serious barrier to proper understanding of the meanings of words and thus of the things the words are meant to signify.[181] Similarly, physicians today spend all their time arguing about an infinite number of trivial matters, instead of learning from experience, to the point that they are always seeking but never finding the truth.[182]

Another related topic is Bacon's preference for simplicity over complexity, a theme he artfully interwove into the language of alchemy. Just as astrology and astronomy were the same for him, so were chemistry and alchemy. Bacon, like many writers on pharmacy in his time, wanted to purify and reduce medicinal substances to their simple essence. The most common way of doing this was by infusion—the way we make tea. This process yielded a very weak form of medicine.[183] But the Arabs wrote about other ways, most notably fermentation and distillation: "The seventh defect [among physicians] is in the fermentation of medicines, because a compound, as Avicenna says, without fermentation will not work." The compound drug must be reduced by proper fermentation into one nature (*unam naturam*) to be effective; "this is the secret of secrets that the common among physicians mistake entirely."[184]

For distillation Bacon also made claims. For instance, he asserted that healing oils and waters ought to be prepared by alchemical means (*per vias alkimie*), through distillations (*per distillationes*). Many medicinal substances are poisonous, like quicksilver, and need to be mitigated. Some, like precious stones, gold, and silver, pass through the body too quickly unless they are dissolved. But if they are prepared through the secret ways of alchemy, with the aid of the *scientia experimentalis*, they can in small quantity help the human body beyond every expectation. Indeed Aristotle affirmed that substances can be reduced to their prime matter (*ad materiam primam*), in the *Metaphysics* and at the end of the *Meteorology*.[185]

Distillation and fermentation, when properly performed, were useful, indeed vital, ways to reduce a medicinal substance to its essential and most powerful nature. What is more, these processes allowed for the virtues of compound drugs to be united into one by ridding each of its extraneous dross. Even a substance as forbidding as vipers' flesh, Bacon argued, could be rendered not only harmless, but useful.[186]

A similar desire for simplicity permeates Bacon's ideas about the healing powers of plants and animals. On this point Bacon contrasted the defects of natural philosophy, which deals with argumentation and universals, with alchemy, which argues from the particular to the primordial generation of things from elements and humors. "Practical" alchemy derives the secret of secrets—how to transmute base metals into gold—of which Aristotle spoke to Alexander, from knowledge about the parts of animals and plants. Similarly, philosophical agriculture (which covered Aristotelian ideas of both botany and zoology) determines through understanding the particulars of plants and animals the nature of the whole and not merely the parts. Unfortunately, alchemy and philosophical agriculture are neglected by students today.[187]

Bacon was anxious to excuse physicians for one fault at least—that they could not practice on their subjects until they got it right because of the "nobility" (*propter nobilitate*) of these subjects. For this reason experience is difficult in medicine.[188] Truth cannot be certified without experience; for that reason, physicians ought to be excused for their huge deficiencies, more than others.[189] Having excused physicians in a rather backhanded way, Bacon renewed his attack on them in the very next paragraph for their discord, and for the sluggishness and death that often follow their procedures.[190] Then he recommended the simplest medicine of all—none. Those who do not use medicines are stronger, more beautiful, and live longer than those who surrender to them,[191] and this is exceedingly plain among northern peoples (*nationibus septentrionalibus*), who seldom use medicines. If physicians understood every medicine and all the nonnaturals (*omnes res non naturales*), and the disposition of the heavens (*dispositionem celi*), then medicines would prolong life and health.[192]

Bacon's last major thematic concern is mathematics, another undergraduate subject he thought crucial to medicine. Throughout his medical works, Bacon was wary of compound medicines, deeming them overpriced, adulterated, ineffective, or even dangerous. Most of the medicines he recommended were simples he associated in the *Opus majus* with the secret of long life: rosemary flowers, the bone in a stag's heart,[193] vipers' flesh, lignum aloes (aloe wood: *Aquilaria agallocha*), opium, deer musk, gold, and Indian rhubarb, with which Bacon had successfully experimented on himself against phlegm.[194] All these substances are rare, and their true nature known only to the most learned philosophers (Bacon offered himself as an example), who described their physical properties and administration at the end of his treatise.

Difficulty arose for the physicians, he asserted, when they tried to compound drugs without the proper knowledge. Latin physicians did not understand the rules of degrees and proportion, which involved many questions Bacon himself found difficult.[195] Alkyndi (al-Kindi) understood what to do, but physicians today are entirely ignorant. Anybody who wants to compound drugs has to be familiar with the agreed principles of mathematics (*communia mathematice*), proportions, and "difficult laws of fractions" (*leges fractionum difficiles*) written about by Alkyndi. What is more, since the skies change every hundred years or so, and therefore their effect on terrestrial beings is different, new calculations need to be made for compound drugs to be effective. But who nowadays knows how to do this? Certainly not a mere physician (*purus medicus*), unless he knows astronomy.[196]

Bacon's point is perhaps less than obvious to modern audiences. Medicine is not independent of other disciplines; in fact, many other things must be mastered before it. There can be no medicine without knowledge of languages; there can be no medicine without proper methods of argumentation; there can be no medicine without alchemy, astrology, philosophical agriculture, and mathematics. Most of all, there can be no medicine without knowledge of natural philosophy: "For Aristotle says that where natural philosophy ends there medicine begins, and the natural philosopher has to supply the first principles of health and infirmity."[197] In other words, a liberal arts education must be propaedeutic to a medical one, or the physician is useless, even dangerous.

By insinuating medicine into learning about Aristotle's natural philosophy Bacon was of course declaring the moral value of a liberal arts education for the physician. The influence of this idea is difficult to judge in England; however, many elite medical patrons employed university-educated physicians without medical degrees. Among many possible examples, Geoffrey Melton, priest and Oxford arts master, attended Mary Bohun, countess of Richmond, Henry IV, Isabella of France, and her husband, Richard II (murdered 1400). Richard II was also advised by priest and arts master John Wyke.[198]

Equally widely shared was Bacon's idea, taken from the *Secretum secretorum*, that the regulation of the nonnaturals through a regimen of health was the proper subject of medical learning. Humanistically minded vernacular poets denounced the fancy potions of the learned physicians as vanity, as did Chaucer in the *Nun's Priest's Tale*, contrasting the temperate regimen of the widow—"Attempree diete was al hir phisik,/And exercise, and hertes suffisaunce"—with the gaudy excesses of Chauntecleer and his meddling medicine-dosing wife Pertelote.[199] Later on, in 1411, the poet Thomas Hoccleve wrote a *Regement of Princes* in English based in part on the *Secretum secretorum* for the future king Henry V.[200] The monk John Lydgate, patronized by Humfrey, duke of Gloucester, wrote a dietary in bad English verse.[201] Numerous translations of the *Secretum* into French and English were made in England during the later Middle Ages and survive into the early printed tradition.[202]

The humanist physician and Oxford chancellor Gilbert Kymer seems to have been Bacon's greatest disciple in the realm of medical alchemy. He led a successful adventure along with other university physicians and a few clerics in 1456 to gain protection from Henry VI to practice the art. Henry's letter patent affirmed, as did Bacon, the reality of occult qualities. It noted that ancient wise men and exceedingly famous philosophers had written secretly about how many glorious medicines could be made from precious stones, oils, plants, and animals, especially the best of all, the Philosopher's Stone, which could be used to treat curable infirmities and prolong human life to its natural extent. It would also transmute metals to gold.[203] The outcome of Kymer's adventure into medical alchemy failed, according to Thomas Norton's *Ordinal of Alchemy* (ca. 1490), but Norton claimed the physician wrote a book on the subject.[204]

A direct chain of "influences" is impossible to outline here, either between Bacon and the vernacular poets or between Bacon and Gilbert Kymer. The most that can be stated is that Bacon was a very early importer of medical humanism from the European continent, whose popularity as an alchemical healer is better documented in the early modern period than during the Middle Ages.[205] Surer indication of the popularity of Bacon's medical works appears in the writings of John Cokkys, Oxford arts master and medical bachelor (d. ca. 1475), who spent his life teaching and practicing medicine in Oxford, apparently with the help of surgeon John Barbour.[206] Cokkys was the author of several medical treatises, including a commentary on Hunayn (Johannitius) titled *Notule M. Johannis de Gallicantu super Johannisium*, found in Bodley MS Ashmole 1475, pages 1–75. He also took an interest in Bacon's alchemical medicine. Bodley MS e musaeo 155 is written in his own hand (save several sections corrected by him) and contains the *Opus tertium*, part of *Opus majus*, the pseudo-Bacon *De retardatione senectutis* (believed by Cokkys to be Bacon's own), *De erroribus medicorum*, and a number of *experimenta*. Most of the extracts concern the medicinal use of alchemical preparations.[207]

Bacon's last major medical work, *Antidotarium*,[208] mentioned *De erroribus* and was probably intended as a fulfillment of sorts of the program its author advanced there.[209] An antidotary is a work about compound medicines, those having more than one ingredient (as opposed to a book of simples, about medicines having only one component); in his, Bacon explored the ways in which simples could be combined usefully. As with Bacon's other medical works, one cannot help but sense Trinitarian philosophical concerns about how various parts can be made into one substance successfully. Fermentation was once again offered as most useful,[210] but what this process was exactly remained a mystery for Bacon. At least he did not describe it to his readers in helpful detail.

Instead, Bacon wrote an often conventional treatise on quantification, reflecting the understanding of Arabic pharmacy as taught at the University of Paris around the middle of the thirteenth century.[211] Following his principal Arabic sources, Avicenna and Haly Abbas, Bacon wrote about the relationship between a medicine's weight and its learned effect. His own system, never clearly worked out, suggested that additional substances be added to the main ingredient of a compound in proportion to its quantity.[212]

Bacon, like Pliny, shrank from what he thought was the ignorant compounding of drugs willy-nilly as irrational and dangerous.[213] Reason and experience should be the guides, and for his rational system Bacon turned to the Greek system of four qualities—hot, cold, moist, and dry—which in a medicine acted against their opposites in the body: "And if a disease against which we are compounding is cold, then a medicine ought to be compounded in quality hot according to the contrary degree of the cold disease."[214] These qualities, according to Galen and other ancient authorities, were divided into four "degrees," with the fourth being the most extreme form. There was also a "temperate" quality, which represented a kind of zero, having a moderating effect.[215]

Bacon accepted this mathematical system as axiomatic, and tried, in a rather half-hearted and ill-tempered way, to show how it might apply to the successful compounding of medicines. He began with one of his favorite metaphors, the plant, its roots, and its branches,[216] to suggest that each compound has at least one, and often more than one, simple "root" (*radix*): "For just as a plant is sustained from its roots, so a compound by its root or roots."[217] This root was a single substance, like vipers' flesh in treacle or aloes in *iera pigra* (a bitter-tasting medicinal paste),[218] which sometimes needed to be combined with others to mitigate its effect, to treat multiple afflictions, or to help carry it to a remote part of the body.[219]

Laxatives and opiates especially caught the author's attention. These were two drugs of great interest to medieval physicians because of their undoubted pharmaceutical effect. But beyond that, laxatives and opiates satisfied their expectations because of these drugs' perceived learned properties. Bacon believed, like most medieval medical thinkers, that illness was a kind of poisoning, and that the job of medical treatment was to purge the body of poison.[220] This interest in poison appears throughout Bacon's medical writings.[221] Vipers' flesh, like many of the best medicines both poisonous and helpful, and the celebrated treacle (*tyriaca*), a universal antidote for poisoning, are mentioned repeatedly in his works.[222]

Opiates are a different story. One might think Bacon's interest in opiates stems from an interest in their soporific quality, and indeed there is some evidence that opium derivatives were used for surgery.[223] Surgery was one of the many medical topics Bacon neglected entirely. His interest was in the fact that opium, being extremely chilling,[224] was able to be compounded with other medicines and prevent them from dissolving before they reached the affected part.[225]

At several turns in the treatise, Bacon repeated his worry that the *moderni* were not getting things right, but his concern that the passing of time had changed the world in important ways went deeper than the somewhat Ciceronian pose the writer chose to strike. Just as the stars were said to have moved from the time of Creation, making new astrological calculations necessary for the physician,[226] so the human body had changed from ancient times, making dosage based on old texts dangerous.[227] Bacon seems to be suggesting that the medicinal substances he dealt with, nearly all of them exceedingly rare,[228] remained immutable in their essential properties throughout the centuries, like the stars. Only the microcosm of humanity changed, requiring constant mathematical recalculations.

Bacon's attempts to separate what was eternal and perfect from what was mutable and imperfect are of course not confined to his medical writings; nor are such concerns limited to Bacon alone. His interest in physicality, food, and the body are striking, but certainly not unique. What is remarkable about Bacon's medical work is the synthetic meaning he drew as much from Scripture as from encyclopedias and scholastic medical texts. His weaving together of the fruit of the Tree of Life from the Old Testament, simple regimen from Pliny, the Philosopher's Stone from pseudo-Aristotle, and precious drugs from Islamic philosophers into a reasonably coherent set of medical theories is an achievement of almost poetic ingenuity, filled with intriguing paradoxes.

Irritating, pompous, and self-important at times, Bacon also managed to convey a sense of wonder and reverence for nature and the works of God no English medical writer would ever surpass. He was able to do this for many reasons, but perhaps more than any because he, like Pliny, conceived a medical system firmly connected to a knowledge of the natural world gained through marvelous books, to which he added his own unshaking conviction of the moral value of the liberal arts. Bacon the encyclopedic medical thinker was a collector and assembler of what he thought was the best medical information, from a variety of sources. As such, his writings represent continuity with the Latin and patristic past, as well as an acceptance of the authority of alien thinkers. What is more, Bacon subordinated medicine to philosophy, making it part of a general knowledge of the nature of the good life and not the property of medical "experts." Like Pliny, he embraced the medicines, but rejected the physicians.

English regimens of health like those admired by Bacon and by vernacular poets were very popular and can be read today in numerous manuscripts and printed copies. Not only do they reveal the popularity of works about the rules of health and behavior in an increasingly courtly English society, but they also may say something about medieval ideas about the nature of kingship itself.[229] Perhaps surprisingly, amidst the struggle for patronage waged by the likes of Hoccleve and Lydgate, only one physician seems to have joined in the fray.[230] Gilbert Kymer compiled his own regimen of health, in Latin, for the humanist Humfrey, duke of Gloucester, youngest son of Henry IV, who made generous gifts of books to Oxford University with Kymer's help in 1439, 1441, and 1443 that formed what is now known as Duke Humphrey's Library.[231] The text's conclusion says it was written on March 6, 1424, in Hainaut, Flanders, where Kymer's patron waged a successful military campaign to win those lands on behalf of his new wife, Jacqueline of Hainaut.[232]

Kymer's regimen suggested regulation of the six nonnaturals, especially food and drink. The document, in a single fifteenth-century manuscript, has twenty-six short chapters, dealing with subjects like selecting bread ("De pane eligendo"),[233] and meats to use and to avoid ("De carnibus vtendis et vitandis").[234] The regimen is exceptional in that Kymer's advice was adapted to Duke Humfrey personally. What is more, the personal advice concerned the most intimate details of Humfrey's sex life: "O illustrious prince . . . your kidneys and genitalia are somewhat debilitated by immoderate frequency of the work of Venus, which the liquidity and scarcity of semen declare."[235] Later on, in chapter 19, Kymer continued along these themes, delivering a virtual sermon on the evils of excessive and improper coitus: "It impedes digestion, suppresses the appetite, causes dryness, corrupts the humors, impoverishes the spirit, chills natural heat, impairs the virtues, suppresses bodily functions, consumes radical moisture, enervates the members, gives rise to evil diseases, effeminizes the sperm, produces lovesickness and jealousy, gives rise to forgetfulness, fatness, neglectfulness, and foolishness, and it shortens the life."[236] All these dire warnings were to no avail, for like many patients, Duke Humfrey defied his doctor, had his first marriage annulled, and married his notorious mistress. But he did give Oxford the books.

CONCLUSION

The medieval English medical text, like the medieval English medical practitioner, defies simple classification. Differences of language, scope of subject matter, level of learning, and philosophical allegiance call into question nearly every explanatory category historians have to offer. Also like the medieval practitioner, the medieval English medical text owes an enormous amount to foreign exemplars, even when it was written in an English vernacular language. To some, this variety could be used to demonstrate the "backward" nature of medieval English medicine, especially as compared to the level of sophistication represented in northern Italian universities. This argument is not without merit, of course, but other explanations are possible. Writers like Gilbert Eagle and Roger Bacon were near contemporaries. Both were clerics and both had strong associations with the Roman papal court. Yet these educated Englishmen produced texts with strikingly different views of the role of the physician and of medicine in general only a few decades apart. This difference indicates not backwardness but hotly debated issues, resolved in the end, very much in Bacon's favor.

Only the medical doctor Gilbert Kymer, in the first half of the fifteenth century, managed to blend humanistic medicine without doctors into the hierarchy implied by the university professorate. He, more than any medieval English physician, gave university medical education the kind of moral, courtly, and intellectual authority it needed to control medical practice for centuries to come. He, more than anyone, saw the value of humanistic, regimen-oriented medicine to potential patrons. Twice chancellor of Oxford University, medical doctor, priest, writer, alchemist, book collector, humanist, first and only rector of the London organization of physicians and surgeons,[237] Gilbert Kymer saw clearly that the success of learned medicine lay with patrons like the duke of Gloucester, who wanted to be educated and read books just like princes did in Italy and France. Duke Humphrey's Library at Oxford University remains today a living testament to the Lancastrian's humanistic aspirations. It also commemorates the man who helped assemble and deliver the books, the duke's physician.

CHAPTER IV

The Institutional and Legal Faces
of English Medicine

THE TWELFTH CENTURY in Europe saw probably the most important development ever to knowledge about healing—the medical university. Before that time learned medicine was taught, along with other forms of dignified learning, in cathedral schools, monasteries, and private establishments. England had two of the oldest universities in the medieval West—Oxford and Cambridge—whose secular and church patrons strove to establish havens of leisure and intellectual sophistication for men studying for the priesthood. These retreats from clerical duty ideally would allow students to be educated to meet increasing demand both for educated parish priests and for learned jurists required by the Crown. Such a system in England left little room to train educated physicians. Oxford and Cambridge had no tradition of medical learning that preexisted the university. This contrasted sharply with the situation in the Italian city-states, for instance. Nor was the Church anxious to have more than a few of the students it supported drawn away from their clerical duties into medical practice. As a consequence, learned medicine was never a strong presence in the medieval English university.

England's large cities had no medical university in the Middle Ages (or for a long time after). This absence of moral and intellectual medical authority, especially in the metropolis of London, presented serious regulation problems for municipal powers. Powerful trade guilds in large cities like York and London policed the practice of their own members and could be called on by city officials to decide about illicit practice among outsiders. But these guilds understandably resented interference by Crown or Church in their prerogatives and resisted attempts to impose the authority of university-educated doctors on the citizenry. Under these conditions, close study of medical learning both within the university and in the legal sphere outside the university can demonstrate much about the tensions and challenges placed on medieval English society as it struggled with the problems of protecting the afflicted and regulating the healers.

MEDICINE AND THE UNIVERSITY

Learned medicine, like Christianity, did not grow on native English soil: it had to be imported from the European continent. Salerno, in southern Italy, was the first medical university in western Europe, and was probably the first university of any kind in the West.[1] It was scarcely typical of medieval universities in general, however, and is best understood as a learned guild of medical practitioners. Indeed by the time Salerno became a university proper in the thirteenth century, it was already near the end of its medical preeminence. Salerno was no doubt dependent on the nearby Benedictine monastery of Monte Cassino for its Latin texts, and is perhaps most famous for the learned medical writer Trota, or Trotula, a woman who studied medicine at the university in the thirteenth century.[2]

Salerno was eclipsed in Italy by the famous medical university of Bologna. Bologna consisted of a doctoral college and a student university, both of which combined the arts and medicine. Very much the poor relation of the wealthy and powerful law faculty, Bolognese physicians nevertheless managed to amass considerable fortunes for themselves. The most notable patron of Bolognese medicine was not the church but the municipality, which found medicine a useful discipline for the health of the city and guarded the medical professorate for its own citizens. Professors were often married laymen rather than clerics. Distinctively, Bologna had no theological faculty until the later fourteenth century.[3]

The model for England's universities was Paris, not Salerno or Bologna, although the last two, along with the medical university of Montpellier,[4] provided texts for Oxford and Cambridge medical study.[5] The medical faculty of the University of Paris, which dates from at least the thirteenth century, consisted of a group of teaching masters. It was, like Cambridge and Oxford, a graduate faculty, in which the undergraduate arts were propaedeutic to medical study, although Paris statutes did provide that medical bachelors could study arts at the same time as medicine.[6]

The graduate faculties of Paris and universities modeled after it as a rule offered doctorates not only in medicine but also in canon and civil law, and in theology, the last of which was considered at such universities to be the ultimate academic degree. At Oxford, for instance, elite fourteenth-century medical doctors like Queen Philippa's physician William of Exeter and university chancellor Adam Tonworth all held double doctorates, with the medical doctorate always preceding the doctorate in theology.[7]

Medicine was never a popular subject at northern European universities during the Middle Ages, and the rationale for including it as a graduate faculty has not yet been explored thoroughly. No doubt Christian thinkers were impressed by the arguments of ancient physicians like Galen about the "professional" status of the medical doctor. Galen denied that medicine was a craft, a charge that annoyed medical doctors throughout the medieval period. Instead, Galen offered that medical practice was not directed toward payment like a craft but instead was given liberally, in a manner indifferent to monetary gain. The doctor could accept an honorarium for his services, but he would never ask for it.[8]

The possibility that medicine could take a place beside the arts, theology, and the laws in a university as a part of godly learning was opened by Christian understanding of ancient physicians like Galen, and by the scriptural commentary of the Roman Church.[9] Arguments like those made by Galen meshed well with Christian scriptural injunctions about charity such as those found in the Gospel of Matthew, in which Jesus gave the disciples power "to heal all manner of sickness and all manner of disease" (Matt. 10:1). He enjoined them to "heal the sick, cleanse the lepers, raise the dead, cast out devils: Freely ye have received; freely give" (Matt. 10:8).[10]

The thoughts of writers like St. Isidore, who asserted that undergraduate disciplines were subordinate to medicine and that medicine was, in fact, a "second philosophy," seem to have held great force in intensely hierarchical universities dominated by clerics, like Paris, Cambridge, and Oxford. Statutes promulgated at Cambridge about 1250 demanded that the medical doctor first graduate in arts.[11] By the fourteenth century at Oxford—whose university records are more complete and detailed for the Middle Ages than those of Cambridge—medicine was firmly established as a graduate faculty, with statutes stipulating the importance of undergraduate arts education to graduate study in medicine.[12] So close were the arts and medical faculties that their forms and procedures were to be written down together without separate sections, and certain arts masters could examine a student if no medical regents could be found.[13]

The closest association between medicine and the arts at the English university was in the medieval science of astrology. In the university, astrology included what we now call astronomy, the two being intellectually inseparable. Astrology was studied in the undergraduate arts faculty as part of the quadrivium, and taught not only the motion of the planets and stars but also their meaning to the world below.[14] Chaucer's fictitious Doctor of Physic could prepare his patients' horoscopes,[15] and many English university physicians were celebrated astrologers. Lewis Caerleon, who was educated at Cambridge and at Oxford, Merton College's Simon Bredon, Oxford chancellor Gilbert Kymer, and John Somerset, who had associations with both Oxford and Cambridge, were among many learned physicians who are known to have studied astrology.[16]

The Persian philosopher-physician Avicenna remarked in his *Canon* that medicine was divided into theory, practice, and empiricism.[17] Medical theory concerned truths that were axiomatic—that there were four humors, for instance—while practice concerned how those truths were put into operation. Empiricism concerned knowledge that was gathered from experience alone, without learned justification. The first two—theory and practice—were taught at the medieval English university. This did not mean that English physicians scorned experience. Cambridge's medical statutes stipulated that the candidate should have practiced medicine for two years before becoming a doctor.[18] A popular commentary on the uroscopy of Giles of Corbeil written by Gilbert Eagle insisted that medicine could not be learned just from books.[19] But even so, it was books with which the university-educated physician began his studies, and books upon which he was examined to achieve his certification.

The prospective medical student began his university education at around the age of fourteen under an experienced master.[20] Especially before the later fifteenth century, the university student in any discipline would have been a cleric, supported by, and educated for, the church. Ideally, he would study the trivium (grammar, rhetoric, logic), the quadrivium (music, geometry, astrology/astronomy, arithmetic), and then the various philosophies. Especially important for the physician were the natural sciences of Aristotle, which taught the student about the operation of the physical universe. He also learned about growth, reproduction, and decay. Then, if form was followed, he would study moral philosophy and metaphysics. By the time he was about twenty, he was a master of arts, and was required to perform two years of regency after that.[21] Students attended lectures at which they took notes, sometimes sitting the same class several times over. They would listen to the disputations or debates of more advanced students and eventually participate in such debates themselves. Their knowledge, as well as their character, was certified by other masters.

Ideally, medical study per se began after the student received his arts education. Both Cambridge and Oxford universities granted the degree of medical bachelor after undergraduate arts study. At Cambridge, the university statutes from the late thirteenth century required three years of study for the medical bachelor, with two years additional if the student had not been regent in arts. As with study in arts, the medical bachelor had to be certified by experienced masters.[22] A similar situation seems to have existed at Oxford, although progress to the baccalaureate is not set down in the statutes. At both universities, the medical baccalaureate seems to have been intended as a university license to practice medicine, rather than a certification to teach medicine like the doctorate.[23]

In fact, very few records remain of the medical baccalaureate being granted at either university before the later fifteenth century. Only three were known to have been given from Oxford throughout the entire fourteenth century, and all of those followed a master of arts. Another was followed by a medical doctorate, and two of the three were followed by doctorates in theology.[24] A study of university-educated medical men indicates that a medical degree was not required for a practitioner to serve as physician to an elite patron, which must have diminished the numbers of men willing to endure the lengthy process of certification. This did not necessarily mean that a physician without a medical degree had never studied medicine in a university, but only that he had not completed formal requirements for a degree.[25] Examples of elite university-educated physicians who had no known medical degrees are numerous. For instance, Geoffrey Melton, priest and Oxford arts master, attended Mary Bohun, countess of Richmond, Henry IV, Isabella of France, and her husband, Richard II.[26] Richard II was also served as physician by priest and arts master John Wyke.[27]

Requirements for the medical doctorate were set out more fully than those for the baccalaureate at Cambridge and Oxford. At Oxford, the student was to hear lectures on medicine for six years; eight if he had not been regent in arts. He was then to perform a series of lectures and disputations, all the while being evaluated by medical regents, who were to attest to his competency and character. Statutes for Cambridge were very similar.[28] The statutes of both universities make special provision for a lack of regents to examine the medical students. Studies of the nature of the student bodies of Cambridge and Oxford confirm the small number of men who studied medicine in the medieval period. At Oxford, for instance, fewer than one-hundred men left any record of medical study. This was about 1 percent of all recorded students.[29] Cambridge's body of medical students was about half the size of Oxford's.[30]

The English doctoral student was examined on several specified texts, based on the writings of Hippocrates and Galen as transmitted to the Latin West via Islamic scholars. At Cambridge, where the list of required readings is more complete than at Oxford, the basis of the medical curriculum was the *Isagoge* of Johannitius, a précis of Galenic medicine.[31] Other texts on diets, urines, prognosis, regimen, and the compounding of drugs were also required. Most of these were based on the medical curriculum called *articella* developed by the masters of the School of Salerno. A similar list of readings was required of Oxford physicians.[32] A study of the book holdings of English physicians shows much wider interests than the required curriculum. John of Gaddesden's *Rosa medicinae* displays an impressive knowledge of medical texts, comprising most of the major authorities of Gaddesden's day, and fellow Mertonian Simon Bredon's unfinished medical text, the *Trifolium*, is also rich in citation.

The greatest problem facing England's medical faculties was the lack of monopoly they or anyone had over the practice of medicine. Oxford physicians had long regulated medical practice within their own precincts, in the same way they had regulated other commercial activity.[33] In other places, most notably London, medicine of every sort was practiced by any number of people, men and women, with only barber-surgery and apothecary trade consistently regulated by a guild structure. In 1421 university physicians, probably led by Gilbert Kymer, tried to remedy this situation by offering themselves up in a petition to Henry V to license medical practitioners. The petition asked that all of England's sheriffs assemble every medical practitioner in the realm at either Oxford or Cambridge, for "trewe and streyte examinacion." Anyone who continued to practice without the license of the university, man or woman, would be subject to fine or imprisonment.[34] If nothing else, such provisions offered legitimacy to physicians who were not clerics, most notably to women, who could not attend English universities. Similar regulation had been put in place by university physicians in Paris,[35] as the petitioners certainly knew, but London was not Paris, and the petition seems to have come to nothing. Perhaps the plan was too ambitious for the universities' tiny medical faculties to implement.

Kymer had a little more success in 1423 by joining forces with wealthy and powerful learned surgeons to form a *comminalte* of physicians and surgeons (known afterward to historians as the Conjoint College of Physicians and Surgeons), on the model of the Inns of Court, to educate and regulate every sort of medical practice.[36] The *comminalte* was to have rooms for reading and disputation; a rector, who would be a university physician; and provision for treating the poor gratis. The object of the petition this time was the lord mayor of the City of London.[37] The *comminalte*, presided over by Kymer as rector, did judge one case. A complainant, one William Forest, charged *comminalte* members with mistreating a hand wound, causing his hand to become disfigured. Kymer offered an astrological explanation of the most learned sort for the unfortunate outcome of Forest's treatment, absolving the surgeons of any blame and saying that the position of the stars and the nature of Forest's body made a bad outcome inevitable. Forest was ordered to maintain silence on the matter.[38] The *comminalte* was not heard from after 1424, probably falling victim to the powerful guild of London barber-surgeons, who must have resented the infringement of their prerogatives by learned physicians from out of town.

By the end of the fifteenth century, the Padua-educated Oxford physician Thomas Linacre and the learned medicine he represented were well on their way to controlling nearly every aspect of elite medical practice just in the way the remarkable Gilbert Kymer and his allies had hoped.[39] Perhaps more than any other social factor, the development of university education led to standardization of medical skills and the establishment of a specialized collection of medical texts in England that a physician had to master. This sort of exclusivity certainly gave the learned physician more power in elite society. But the exclusion of women, Jews, and, after the time of Henry VIII, non-Anglicans once again drove many of the best would-be medical students abroad and created even more problems for foreigners wanting to practice in England.[40]

LAW AND MEDICINE

Oxford and Cambridge concerned themselves with many other types of business apart from the education of physicians, who were, in any case, a small part of the university community before the fifteenth century. And yet, the way in which learned medicine developed was shaped in large part by the nature of the institution of the university as a whole, where medicine found a home. The same is true for the medical aspects of the law. The Romans left behind traces of their law, as did the Celts. Anglo-Saxon invaders brought with them the laws of their Germanic fellow tribesmen. The Normans reintroduced Roman law in the eleventh century, which reconciled with that of the Anglo-Saxons. Canon law, the law of the Roman Catholic Church, was present in England from the time of the Christian missionaries. Bodies of precedent developed and innovation became necessary as population grew and bureaucracies became more complex.[41]

Medical matters were a part of all this, but not a very large part. Even so, legal records contain endless bits and pieces of evidence for society's notions about health and disease, the causes of death, the ways people suffered injuries, the words used to describe disease, and the way medical practitioners were valued. This evidence is difficult to organize, scattered in many different sources, and changes very little through time. Arguments about what it all means are difficult to advance under such circumstances. But the fact remains that these scattered fragments of information give a kind of vividness to matters of life, disease, and death missing from every other source of medical evidence.

The interaction between medieval English law and medical matters can be viewed from at least two standpoints: the relatively rare instances when a medical practitioner is a party in some legal proceeding, and the much more common situation when a party suffering some physical injury or death comes under lay judgment. Understandably, medical historians have tended to emphasize legal cases in which practitioners are charged with wrongdoing, sometimes using the legally anachronistic term "malpractice" to describe these encounters.[42] In fact, laws relating to medical practice before the early modern period were underdeveloped: only within university towns and among members of guilds were standards of practice well established.[43]

Legal handbooks do give some hints of how judges were to make decisions concerning medical practitioners, but the body of precedent is not
detailed and seems to be based not on English custom but on canon law.[44]
This type of law, like the structure of the university, was imported from
the Continent. The Anglo-Norman *Mirror of Justices*, written about 1290,
touched on medicine by and large only to help a judge determine whether
a medical practitioner had committed homicide or mayhem:

> Physicians [*fisciens*] and surgeons being learned in their faculties and prov-
> ably making lawful cures, and having clear consciences, so that in nothing
> have they failed their patients that to their art belongs, if their patients die,
> are not homicides or mayhemers; but if they undertake to make a cure which
> they do not know how to bring to a successful end, or, although they have
> such knowledge, they behave stupidly or negligently, as by applying heat
> instead of cold, or the reverse, or too little of the cure, or if they do not
> apply a due diligence, more especially in their cauterisings and amputations,
> which are things that cannot lawfully be done save at the peril of the prac-
> titioners, then, if their patients die or lose a limb, they are homicides or
> mayhemers.[45]

Significantly, there was no instruction as to how to determine whether a
person actually was a physician or surgeon, nor was there any provision for
expert medical testimony.

An illustration of the typical interest of the law in the actions of a medical
practitioner can be found in the records of the Sheriff's Court of John
Preston, sheriff of London.[46] In a case dated 29 August 1320, Alice of Stocking complained that on 10 June 1320 the defendant, John of Cornhill,
surgeon (*surigicus*), approached her on Fleet Street, London, and said he
could cure her of a malady of the feet (*infirmitate in pedibus*) in fifteen days
for half a mark (a mark was 13 shillings, 4 pence, or two-thirds of a pound).
Instead, as a result of John's treatment, within six days Alice was unable to
put her feet to the ground and became incurable. On 23 June 1320, Alice
complained, John broke into her house with force and arms, against the
king's peace, and stole items worth 20 shillings and otherwise damaged her
in the amount of 100 marks. On 2 September 1320, a jury found for the
plaintiff, awarding her damages of £30 16s. 8d., somewhat less than what
she had requested but among the largest recorded in the rolls of this particular court.

The formulas "force and arms" and "against the king's peace" define
trespass in this period, and the issue here clearly is that.[47] By the 1360s
the law of trespass had grown more complex, and prosecutions of medical
practitioners for undertaking to cure (*assumpsit*) and instead making matters worse began to be recorded. These actions appear in the context of
claims thought to be similar, for instance, of a handler allowing grain or

livestock to deteriorate under his care, or acting negligently when goods like wool were handed over for improvement.[48]

Coroners' rolls, like legal handbooks or court records, preserve a wealth of detail about how people, otherwise unknown, lived and died. The coroner's job was to investigate injuries or deaths that were in any way unusual.[49] Several coroners' rolls survive in which inquests are presented according to a formula: "On such and such a day the Coroner and Sheriff are informed that an individual is lying dead of a death other than his or her rightful death in such and such place; and thereupon they proceed thither and having summoned a jury they diligently inquire what happened." Those having knowledge about the deceased were included in the jury, which then reported as to the cause of death: felony or misadventure. The *Mirror of Justices* directed the coroner to confer with "good folk" as to the manner of the killing, "if from misadventure, whether it came from God or man; if from famine, whether from poverty or from common pestilence." Other possible causes were suggested, including "horse, cart, mill, sails or wheels of a mill." Tournaments, jousts, medleys, and other dangerous sports were special cases "forasmuch as such sports are dangerous, everyone ought to prepare himself so that God may find him in a holy life." The ancient custom of the coroner's holding views in cases of "sodomy, and on infant monsters who had nothing of humanity, or had more of the beast than man in them" had died out, the writer said, due to the general decrease in those consequences of sinfulness that had taken place in recent times.[50] *Fleta*, another late-thirteenth-century legal formulary, stipulated that in the case of death by mischance, those who drowned, died suddenly, or were crushed had to be viewed naked.[51]

The catalog of murder and mayhem recorded in these documents leads one to believe that drunkenness and violence were daily spectacles. Almost any excuse seemed to serve to revive an old quarrel or begin a new one. London's Lucy Faukes in 1322 was murdered by a husband and wife, old friends who picked a fight with her so they could kill her and steal her clothes.[52] Walter de Elmeleye died in 1301 as the result of a brawl begun when Alice Quernbetere, being drunk, engaged in "wordy strife" with two workmen, calling them "tredekeiles."[53]

Indeed drunkenness figures prominently as a contributing factor in many deaths. John de Markeby, goldsmith, in 1339 "was drunk and leaping about" in a friend's house "where he accidently wounded himself with a knife called a 'Trenchour de Parom' (the instrument of death was characteristically described in detail—this one was probably used in leatherwork) that hung on his belt, inflicting a mortal wound in his left leg above the knee 5 inches deep and 3 inches broad of which he died the same night."[54] In 1300 Richard le Brewer was carrying a bag of malt and, overcome by drink, stumbled, rupturing his bowels and diaphragm, and so he lived for two days, dying about the hour of curfew.[55] William Bonefaunt, skinner, stood "drunk, naked, and alone at the top of a stair . . . for the purpose of relieving nature when by accident he fell headforemost to the ground and forthwith died."[56]

Drowning claimed an extremely large number of victims; witness one John Gabb, who, asleep while leaning on a willow tree, fell into a creek and drowned.[57] William Wombe, a cleaner of latrines, entered the river Thames to bathe in 1339 and drowned.[58] Especially common were the drownings of children, and parental neglect is often cited as a contributing cause.[59] A coroner's roll of 1267 reported that a three-and-a-half-year-old child fell into a ditch and drowned while his mother went out for beer,[60] whereas another infant drowned at 9 A.M. on 8 April 1268 while his parents were in church.[61] One court instructed that, in the case of drowning, the coroner could order that a pond be filled in.[62]

Fire or burning were commonly cited causes of death, especially in urban areas. In an unusual case, Alice Ryvet died in 1326 when she accidentally set her home and shop on fire late at night with a candle. She and her husband escaped, but he was so enraged at her carelessness that he pushed her back into the flames and fled. Alice died of her burns.[63]

A roll of an eyre of 1218–19 in which the king's justices heard the results of coroners' inquests, among other things, gives a statistically invalid but nonetheless interesting catalog of mortality: 3 people were crushed by carts, 1 fell on an axe, 1 suffocated in his bed from immoderate drinking, 64 died of drowning, 1 fell on his own arrows, 23 fell from their horses and drowned, 2 fell from carts and drowned, 1 fell from a ship, 1 (a two-year-old girl) drowned in a ditch, 4 fell from horses, 1 fell from a horse onto his own knife, 1 fell from a horse into a pile of hog food, 1 fell from an oak tree, 1 fell from a grange (granary), 1 fell on the ice and drowned, 2 fell into vats of molten lead, 1 fell on a scythe, 1 was crushed by a falling door, 1 fell off a haystack, 1 was crushed by an oak tree, 1 was crushed by a falling wall, 6 were crushed by mill wheels, 4 died in the woods, 1 died from a pig bite, 1 died from cold and snow, 2 died from cold in the field, 1 died from cold in the woods, 2 died of sickness, 8 were found dead in a field (including a boy found dead in a field in a chest),[64] 1 committed suicide by hanging, and 5 died of undetermined causes.[65]

A unique inquest into the death of a large number of persons took place in 1322 in London when "a great multitude of poor people were assembled at the gate of the Friars Preachers seeking alms." Fifty-five people were crushed during the distribution of the estate of Henry Fingrie, fishmonger and former sheriff of London.[66]

The act of elimination was notably fraught with peril, as the coroners' rolls attest. John le Stolere, "a pauper and mendicant of the age of 7 years," was run down in the street by a twelve-year-old cart driver while he was "relieving nature."[67] A fight arising from the casting of the contents of a urinal into a stranger's shoe claimed one Philip de Asshendone in 1322,[68] and an unfortunate Richard le Rakiere, seated on a latrine in his house, was drowned when the planks gave way.[69]

The reader may well remark on the detail with which wounds—which the victims seemed glad to display in open court if they could—were measured, in inches or by the number of bones that had to be extracted from them. For example, a coroner's roll of 1271 reported that John of Bordelais was struck "wickedly and feloniously" with a sword "between the parting of the hair and the ear; . . . inflicting upon him a big wound which was five inches long, three inches wide, and which extended downward as far as the brain, so that thirteen pieces of bone were extracted."[70] These descriptions are relics of an earlier time when the victim was compensated by the size and location of the wound and some concrete measure was needed: a twelfth-century custom book stipulated 4d. for every inch of the wound in an exposed part and 8d. for every inch in a covered part, and that the victim ought to be reimbursed for any cost he had to pay in the healing of the wound.[71]

Lay judgment was considered sufficient in these inquests. The ability of the layperson to make medical decisions was in fact the rule rather than the exception. One example is the so-called essoin of bed sickness, in which an ill person was officially excused from some legal obligation. The usual process involved "4 knights of the shire" visiting the sick person to determine if he actually was sick, and how long he was expected to remain so. Unfortunately, the nature of the illness was not specified, and it was standard to allow a year and a day from the viewing for the man to recover. This system presented some difficulties, as a recovered person could be required to remain in bed for the remainder of the year.[72]

The expert medical witness was rare in late medieval England, but there are a few rather ambiguous examples. The name of a barber or surgeon does come up in coroners' rolls as a witness, as in the case of the death of Christina Morel (1300), who was said to have died from a kick in the stomach during a fight. Master William the surgeon was summoned as a neighbor to tell what he knew. But there is no indication he acted in any expert capacity, only that he happened to live nearby.[73]

The Coram Rege Rolls, which recorded cases before the king's justices, chronicled a dispute in 1283 between an abbot from the Isle of Wight and a countess Isabella de Forz, who, the abbot claimed, sent some men in her charge to attack his monks "to the manifest contempt of the lord king." Isabella answered that her men had been stationed on the island to keep the peace and had been attacked by a band of armed monks, who shot a horse and several men. The county coroner was ordered to come and view the men and their wounds, and reported that some would die, especially one who had been shot by an arrow in the chest. He instructed the bailiffs to detain the man responsible until the outcome of the wounds had been determined. The bailiff subsequently seized the monks, along with horses, hauberks, habergeons, haketons, iron gloves, lances, swords, and shields. The bailiffs were subsequently asked how they knew they had the right to hold these men. They replied that the coroner, who was there with a jury, caused the arrow to be drawn from the wound in the presence of some of them. Moreover, one of the most reputable surgeons in those parts was sent for to examine the wounded men. He said he did not believe that the man who had been struck in the chest could escape with his life.[74]

An entry dated 1300 in the rolls of the London mayor's court gives us another early example. William, rector of the Church of St. Margaret Lothebury, was summoned for claiming four putrid wolves sent from abroad in a barrel. The defendant said that he bought the wolves because of a disease he had called "le lou." The defendant admitted to the mayor and aldermen that he was not suffering from this disease, nor did he know anybody who was, and that he was not a physician or a surgeon. He was handed over to the sheriffs, for having claimed falsely that he had the disease, until the truth of the matter could be known. The sheriffs were ordered to summon all the physicians and surgeons of London, who came into court and said that they could not find in any of their medical or surgical writings any disease against which the flesh of wolves could be used.[75]

Another use the law made of medical practitioners was to help prevent the spread of disease. The City of London appointed recognized experts to bar diseased persons from entering through the city gates (London then was surrounded by walls) or entering its prisons or baths (baths implied brothels, also called stews). These persons were typically barbers, who were trained to recognize visible signs of illness.[76] In these cases, the city officials seemed to fear the spread of leprosy, which would have been visible on the skin. In another case, in 1354, the mayor of London summoned the surgeons of the city to say whether an apothecary, John le Spicer of Cornhill, had treated a jaw wound correctly.[77]

References to disease in medieval legal documents are most often made incidentally to other matters, but they occur often enough to give some notion about lay understanding of medical matters and vocabulary. The falling sickness is the most frequently cited cause of death when disease is mentioned and the term seems to cover any sort of sudden death.[78] John Bristow in 1300 went to the church to pray and, seized with the falling sickness (*morbo caduco*), placed himself near a pillar and died.[79] On 30 June 1267, Reginald Stead, went out into the meadows of Eaton belonging to his lord "and had the falling sickness [*morbum caducum*] and died at once."[80]

The disease was not always fatal; a man in 1221 begged to be excused from fighting a duel because he had the falling sickness.[81]

Other sorts of illnesses are mentioned far less frequently. "Mau del flaunke" (pain in the abdomen) struck down one Simon as he was about to milk a cow on 18 July 1271,[82] and in 1301 "tisik" (phthisis) carried off Roger le Brewer at the home of a friend before a priest could arrive. In the same year quinsy was responsible for the death of Richard of St. Albans, who "grievously suffering from a quinsy [morbo squinacie], wandered about and entered his master's stable where he fell down and suddenly died." The corpse was viewed, the neck and throat of which appeared large and swollen.[83] An excited bystander at a game called "le wrastleng" (wrestling) shot contestant Thomas Clark with an arrow at Isham in 1309. Clark recovered, but later died of "le flux." The jury decided that the disease did not occur as a consequence of the wound.[84] Another man suffered a similar fate in 1266. He was wounded, recovered, and then died of "fluxus ventris" (diarrhea). The jury decided as it had in the previous case.[85] A stroke of paralysis (morbus paraliticus) carried off a man in 1301 following a slight head injury,[86] and bad air killed one John de Maldone in 1301 while he was cleaning a well.[87] On 11 June 1301 Robert le Braceour spent the night asleep outside the church of St. Bartholomew the Little, after a drunken brawl, and died at the house of a friend several days later, the jury decided, "from the illness he contracted by passing the night in the street."[88] William Hampnie in 1300 had suffered from a malady in his leg called a "festre" for three years, and on "Sunday about the hour of Vespers, a certain vein in his leg burst, so that, being unable to stop the flow of blood, he became weakened and lingered until the hour of curfew when he died."[89] A child who did not follow his surgeon's advice for treatment of "pin and web" (an eye disease) occasioned a suit in Chancery to defend the surgeon's reputation,[90] whereas a cure for baldness that went wrong caused the victim to sue his barber for breaking a covenant in 1288.[91] An acute fever (febre acuta) was said to have rendered a man impotent, according to the Coram Rege Rolls of 1294,[92] and a quartan fever in 1301 killed William de Ottefored, who, "grievously suffering," asked to be allowed to rest at the house of William Mokelyn until the attack passed off. He lay on the ground, and after a while he died.[93] Thomas Birchester charged negligence against one Lewis the Leech (leche), Lombard, who had undertaken (assumpsisset) in Southwark for a suitable fee to cure Thomas of an injury of the kidneys near his privy parts and under the skin of his body ("de quadam lesione in le reynes iuxta membra sua infra pellem corporis sui").[94]

The London Eyre of 1276 reported the bizarre case of an accidental poisoning. Andrew le Sarazin, who was suffering from a fever, consulted Master John de Hexham and his brother, both doctors. John sent Master William de Crek to give Andrew pills. Later Andrew and his valet Richard ate such a quantity of the pills that they died soon after. The doctors were cleared of homicide.[95]

The death of a friendless felon in prison could be the subject of an inquest. William Cook was arrested for stealing a horse and later died in prison on Saturday, 1 August 1322, "of hunger, thirst, and privation",[96] and Newgate Prison claimed William de Brich and Thomas atte Grene in 1322.[97] Advanced age was sometimes cited as a contributing factor in a death. Alice le Pusere in 1326 wanted to descend the stairs from a solar (upstairs bedroom); "being of the age of 80 years and more, she accidentally fell from the top to the bottom, and was carried by her friends into the solar where she had her ecclesiastical rights" and died.[98]

Reports of suicide, almost always by hanging or by drowning, are numerous, and very often are said to result from some sort of named mental distress.[99] Isabella, wife of Robert de Pampesworth of Breadstreet, London, had suffered long from a disease called "frensy" and, alone in her chamber at the hour of Prime (about 6:00 A.M.), while her son's servant went to the kitchen to get her some food, hanged herself "while suffering from the aforesaid disease."[100] In 1398 Edith Rogers of Wick, who was demented or insane (*demens et insans*), drowned in a well through her own negligence and insanity.[101] In 1320 one Joan, who was mad (*arage*), drowned herself in the Thames. The king did not exercise his right to confiscate in case of suicide, as the jury judged her mad. Her goods were given in alms for her soul.[102] The Crown dealt similarly with Alice de Warewyk, who, while staying with friends, as she had been *non compos mentis* for half a year, ran into the street in a wild state and threw herself into the Thames in February 1340.[103] John de Irlaund hanged himself with his shirt in 1322 and, in spite of attempts to resuscitate him, died.[104] One Richard, a madman (*freneticus*), stabbed himself in the stomach and died three days later,[105] whereas Roger of Tadcourt Yorkshire in 1219 "arose in the night and drowned himself."[106]

The disposal of the property of suicides presented a problem for medieval jurists. *Fleta* stated:

> Just as a man may commit felony in slaying another, so he may in slaying himself; for if one who has lately slain a man or has committed some like act whence felonies arise, conscious of his crime and in fear of judgement, slays himself in any fashion, his goods accrue to the Crown. . . . But should anyone slay himself in weariness of life (*tedio vite*) or because he is unable to support some bodily pain, he shall have his son as his heir. . . . Similarly madmen (*furiosi*) and those who are frenzied (*frenetici*), childish (*infantuli*), deranged (*mente capti*) or are suffering from a high fever, although they kill themselves, do not commit felony or forfeit their inheritances because they lack sense and reason.[107]

The *Mirror of Justices* distinguished between different kinds of mental problems. "As to madmen (*arragez*), we must distinguish; for those who are frantic or lunatic (*les frenetics e les lunatics*) can sin feloniously, and thus may sometimes be accountable, . . . but not those who are continually mad (*continuelement arragez*)."[108] There also seems to have been a distinction made between those who could not be held accountable for their actions because of their age or intelligence. "As to fools (*fous*) let us distinguish, for all fools can be adjudged homicides except natural fools (*foux nastres*) and children within the age of 7 years; for there can be no crime or sin without a corrupt will (*corrupcion de volunte*) and there can be no corruption of will where there is no discretion and an innocent conscience."[109]

Examples of these principles in practice are common. In one case heard before the Crown in 1212, the king was asked to be consulted about an insane man who was in prison and, because of his madness, claimed to be a thief when he was not.[110] In 1225 a jury found Richard of Brent not guilty of larceny. The jurors did not suspect him of any theft, "save a fowl which he took in his madness at the time when he was a lunatic (*in furore tempore quo fuit lunaticus*)."[111] In 1298 a jury was asked to decide on a case in which Johanna de Pontefract was claimed to have been illegally dispossessed of property "while she was laid up with a serious illness so that she was out of her mind (*quod inmemor sui fuit*)."[112]

Practical instructions for handling insane people (*de hominibus dementibus*) are given in a borough customs book of 1344, directing that "the mayor shall take their goods and chattels and deliver them to the next of kin to be kept until they are restored to sanity. And the next of kin must provide a guardian for the bodies of such insane persons," for their own protection and those around them.[113] The Borough Customs of Hereford in 1486 stated that, in case a person involved in a transfer of property was suspected to be mentally unsound, the bailiff should examine those nearest to the person and, if necessary for the person's own protection, appoint a guardian.[114]

Civil courts tended to deal with those suspected of practicing magic. In 1371 John Crok was instructed by the king's justices to produce a bag with a dead man's head in it. John produced the bag. He said the head was that of a Saracen and he had bought it in Toledo, Spain, in order to house a spirit in it so that the said spirit would answer questions. The book also contained in the bag had experiments (*experimentis*) written on it. John claimed he had not done anything with the head or the book yet, and the bag and its contents were burned before the king at Westminster. John was ordered to swear on the gospel not to do anything else contrary to faith.[115]

In 1365 Nicolas, a clerk of Southwark, was summoned to answer Richard, son of Nicholas Cook. It was charged that Nicholas seized Richard and imprisoned him until Richard "lost his senses at the sight of the evil spirits raised by the diabolical conjurations" made by Nicholas to the loss of £100. Nicholas in turn claimed he was only trying to teach the boy to read and sing as he did with other boys. He had to pay damages to Richard's father of 20 marks.[116]

Leprosy and plague are two special categories of disease that present themselves as particularly important to the Middle Ages. A case in the plea and memoranda rolls of London in 1408 gives some idea of the fear the former could excite in a sufferer.[117] A leech swindled John Clotes out of jewels worth 9 marks, gold worth 60s., and a sword worth 6s. 8d., by claiming he had an infallible cure for leprosy,[118] and in 1385, having been raped by a leper called Adam, a servant named Margaret "became hysterical by reason of shame, the rape, and the aforesaid Adam's disease, that she at once went out of her mind" and died shortly thereafter.[119] A St. Ives fair court on 28 April 1287 decided that Ralph Keyse had received lepers in a house, to his neighbors' and to merchants' great peril. He was fined 6d.[120]

Local courts on occasion found it necessary to declare people lepers. For example, in a Norwich leet roll (record of a manor court) of 1374–75, Thomas Tylel, weaver, was declared a leper "who must go out [of the city]" and declared Richard Jobbe, lodged in a house at Normanspital, to be a leper also.[121]

A Coram Rege Roll of 1420 reported that Henry IV, exercising protection of public health, complained to the sheriff of Lincoln saying he had heard that John Louth of Boston, mercer, "is a leper and commonly mingles with the men of the aforesaid town and communicates with them in public as well as private places and refuses to move himself to a place of solitude [*ad locum solitarium*], as is customary . . . to the serious danger of the aforesaid men and their manifest peril on account of the contagious nature of the disease [*propter contagionem morbi*]." The sheriff was to take men who knew John and had information about the disease, see if he was a leper, and, if so, isolate him.[122]

In 1291 a jury in Norfolk was asked to investigate a leper house founded by the famous justice Ralph Glanville and his wife, Bertha. In a tone of extreme disapproval, they reported that of the ten lepers in the house, four were healthy and did not need to be held, and that they had had no chaplain for a long time. All were forced to swear that they would never leave the house or climb the trees to chat with friends. They were forbidden to complain, with or without justification, but had to be grateful for everything that was done for them. The manager, the jurors concluded, kept "a strong and massive dog" in front of the door, to keep friends and family from asking about the inmates or getting to know the conditions there.[123]

The serious disruptions caused by plague, which began in England in 1348,[124] affected every aspect of medieval life. This is reflected in legal documents. For example, a Lincolnshire town in 1375 complained that it was in danger of becoming a marsh, because, after the first plague, "the lands of the township have become so alienated and divided that the keepers of the ditches know not by whom they should be repaired."[125] River traffic also was disrupted, as a complaint before the king's justices in Norfolk in 1360 shows. The river Smallee became blocked through no one's fault because "the river fell out of use at the time of the pestilence and nothing was carried on it so that weeds continually grew in it from that time until the present time," and no one could remember who cleaned it last.[126] Recurrences of the plague in 1407 and 1420 caused the royal courts to be adjourned in London.[127]

The Coram Rege Rolls of 1356 in Hereford show the effect of the labor shortages plague caused, and reaction to various laws passed to keep workers from demanding higher wages. It was alleged that Robert Gerard, vicar of Aldbury Church, and Richard of Fulham, hermit "scorned and poured contempt day after day on the king's statute and ordinance of labourers, artisans, and servants, made by the said king and his council for the common utility of the realm of England, publicly preaching and proclaiming that there is no statute that would restrict labourers, artisans and servants from taking for their labour and services as much as they pleased to take ... and that if, it was ordained or decreed otherwise, the said statute and ordinance were falsely and wickedly made." The two "publicly and openly propounded these wicked things, setting a dangerous example ... whereby [the people] are more rebellious and bolder in their outrages and trespasses." The vicar and his friend were dealt with mildly, being found guilty only of "traipsing round the countryside."[128]

Occasionally records disclosed where a sick or injured person went for care or how the sick were cared for. Many seem to have come to London for treatment. In 1300 William Wattepas, who had long lived in Essex, came to London to be cured of a wound in his arm. He was taken ill in Billingsgate and died there, jurors said, not of the wound.[129] In 1325, on the Sunday before Palm Sunday (31 March), Thomas de Hodesdone of Herefordshire was wounded in a fight with a neighbor, who struck him on the top of the head, "inflicting a mortal wound 4 1/2 inches long and penetrating the brain." Thomas was taken by friends to London for medical treatment and died the following Tuesday at nightfall.[130]

Doctors did make house calls. A certain Simon the Monk, *physicus* in 1218 went to the house of William le Vacheur with nine other men, killed William, and burned down his house, because William had revealed the affair Simon was having with a patient to whose house "he went many times to cure her."[131] Very occasionally was an injured person cared for in an institution, and there is no evidence that this care involved any specialized treatment. Philip de Assendone, who was struck in the head with a staff in an argument, "was thence carried by men unknown for charity's sake" to the Hospital of St. Mary without Bishopsgate, where he died several days later.[132]

The law afforded special protection to women during the medieval period, and rape was one of the few crimes a woman could prosecute herself. Beliefs about conception and gestation are preserved in these cases. One Joan in 1313 produced her child as evidence against her rapist. "It was said that this was a wonderful thing, for that a child could not be engendered without the consent of both parties." The attacker was freed.[133] The fact that a childless woman would almost certainly lose her property on the death of her husband to a male relative seems to have occasioned a number of "posthumous pregnancies." The claim by one such woman that her son was his late father's heir was overturned by a jury in 1294 because the child's birth had occurred forty weeks and eleven days after the husband's death, which was 11 days past the legal limit.[134] *Fleta* advised women who claimed they were pregnant after a husband's death to be examined by "lawful and discreet women" (*legales et discretas mulieres*) and thereafter isolated.[135] *Fleta* also outlined legal policy in abortion, stating that a man who had intercourse with a pregnant woman, gave her poison, or struck her in the belly to procure abortion or prevent conception, "if the feotus was already formed and quickened," committed homicide. "A woman also commits homicide if, by a potion or the like, she destroys a quickened child in her womb."[136]

Matters affecting public health appeared with increasing frequency in these documents as time went on. The isolation of lepers has already been mentioned, and there are numerous examples of other attempts to control nuisances and health hazards. For instance, an account from the Coram Rege Rolls of 1293 stated that Edward I had directed the sheriff of Oxford to investigate the contamination of bread and ale by water taken from places that "are disgraceful and dirty on account of the filth." Also, taverns were accused of having "mixed, putrid and corrupt wines, . . . whereby some who buy them incur serious maladies and often some of them sustain death." The sheriff was instructed that he must taste these wines at intervals, to assure their quality. The king further complained that people keep certain animals in their houses, put dung in the streets, "and by it the air there is infected and corrupted to the serious damage and peril of loss of life, not only of the clerks but also of the laymen."[137] In another case, a leet roll of 1390 in Norwich fined a barber 12d. because he was "wont to throw putrid blood into the king's highway in abominable offence."[138]

Generalizations are difficult to draw from such a welter of evidence. Legal records of prosecutions almost by definition do not chronicle the normal, whether in medical practice or in other matters. What is more, in a time during which laws of trespass and contract were only just developing, and during which standards of medical practice were hardly established or separated from other types of standards of public conduct, little in the way of a pattern emerges. Still, a few conclusions can be drawn from this type of testimony.

The most obvious aspect of medical involvement in the legal sphere is the importance of lay judgment. Men of good character formed a jury, and unlike today, these were ideally men who had personal knowledge of the parties involved. Medical "experts" were nearly unknown, or, at least, they had no more specialized expertise than any other sort of tradesperson called in to give an opinion. Interestingly enough, practically the only sort of medically related expertise regularly sought by courts was that of women, who rendered opinions in cases of pregnancy and impotence.

There is also the occasional recognition that a medical practitioner, exercising "due diligence," was to a certain extent protected from the same sort of legal liability that a layperson would be. Reputation, as in nearly every other medical matter, was of vital importance here. Obviously, if a person was widely known in the community as a good surgeon, then he or she could practice surgery with some sort of special legal protection. As the Forest case demonstrates, however, the surgeon's reputation could be menaced by a bad outcome. Gilbert Kymer, armed with the learned judgment and reasons a university education could afford, offered a certain amount of protection to the surgeon in the Forest case, but the failure of the *comminalte* demonstrates the lack of strong social sanction for such protection.

Next, English law by its very nature required certain standards by which it could exact recompense, for no other reason than fairness. It may seem odd to fine an assailant according to the number of bones extracted from a wound or the number of inches deep or long it measured, but this method was probably as equitable as any. Medieval English law developed certain standards of medical judgment and employed medical vocabulary out of the necessity to preserve social order and dispense justice fairly. What is important about the English Middle Ages is that this was done for the most part by laypeople.

Finally, the use by municipalities of guilds and guildlike organizations such as the *comminalte* to exercise social control is striking. Scholars have tended to view guilds as fraternal organizations that trained craftspersons and promoted trade. In other words, guilds of every sort historically have been considered as economic entities. Clearly by the late fifteenth century the barber-surgeons, who were well-represented in larger cities like York and London, were training apprentices[139] and had achieved stability and recognition.[140]

Increasingly, however, the guild has been viewed as a means for municipal authorities to exert control and establish hierarchy in towns and cities.[141] Certainly Gilbert Kymer's *comminalte*, which arranged physicians

and the surgical crafts in a strict hierarchy and exerted, briefly, quasi-judi-
cial authority over the London citizenry, would be a good example of a
guildlike structure exerting such control. Other historians have shown that
one of the most common functions of guilds and guildlike structures was
to exclude women from the most gainful forms of independent employment.[142] Medical practice presents a modest exception to this exclusion.
Women could not study at universities, which barred them from the most
elite level of practice. There was no provision for them, or for midwifery
practice, in the *comminalte*. But on levels of practice not dominated by the
priesthood, women's presence was recognized, although women did not
appear in positions of much power.

The 1381 poll tax of the London suburb of Southwark, which stated the
occupations of every householder, noted 1 woman barber and 1 woman
midwife out of 137 women householders listed (by comparison, there was
1 woman carpenter, 1 woman mason, and many, many more engaged in
occupations related to food and textile production).[143] No evidence that
either of these women was a guild member survives, and it is likely they
practiced their trade independently. But of all the York craft guilds only
the ordinances of the guild of barber-surgeons from the late fourteenth
century allowed women to be apprentices.[144]

London did not make such provisions, but there were other forms of
recognition of women's importance to medical practice. In 1368 the mayor
and aldermen of the City of London swore four master surgeons to police
their craft, to ensure reasonable fees were charged, and to report to the
mayor and aldermen on these and other related matters. By 1389 another
admission had taken place, this time charging the masters to oversee both
men and women practicing surgery.[145] Later the Physicians' Petition of
1421 provided for women practicing medicine to be examined along with
men.

The university and the municipality, as bodies that oversaw medical practitioners, acted to enable some groups to exercise their trade or profession.
Sometimes, as in the case of the Physicians' Petition or the *comminalte*,
Crown, university, and municipality even cooperated to control practice.
They also acted to establish certain standards of good practice, with very
limited success in the medieval period. And, in the case of legal authority,
governments used the law and the organizations they permitted that were
subject to the law to preserve order and to protect the citizenry. The limits
of proper medical practice, the question of who should be a practitioner,
and what he or she could be expected to know were still very much open
even in the late fifteenth century.

CHAPTER V

Well-Being without Doctors:
Medicine, Faith, and Economy among
the Rich and Poor

TODAY people in developed countries have high expectations from scientific medicine and from the professionals and institutions that deliver it. Advances in public health, medicine, surgery, and related fields give wealthier people at least the hope that medicine will restore good health and prolong life. And rightly so—the state of modern scientific medicine would have been almost unimaginable even fifty years ago. Also understandable is the way medical historians have looked to the university-educated physician as the ancestor of today's scientific medical practitioner. This point of view is well justified in that mastery of a set body of texts, which university education demanded of the medieval physician, remains the backbone of medical training.

It may surprising, then, that medieval English people were far from agreement that learned medicine was an important or even desirable service. Most were too poor even to dream of visiting a medical practitioner, but some who were rich enough avoided doctors by choice. Many of medieval England's social elite advocated pathways to well-being without resort to "professional" medical practitioners. At the other end of the social scale, the poor, the friendless, the elderly, and the chronically ill had no choice but to rely on Christian charity, which was concerned with the more pressing matters of food, shelter, and spiritual comfort than with what seemed like minor complaints. The social elite and the dispensers and recipients of Christian charity shared similar notions about well-being. Both groups stressed sound diet, frugal living, and attention to spiritual matters over bodily concerns.

The tradition of Roman Stoicism, based in large part on the writings of Pliny, informed the notions of well-being held by many medieval English people. Roger Bacon cited Pliny frequently on matters of health and, tying his arguments to Holy Scripture, reminded his readers how humanity's first sin was not so much disobedience but eating the wrong thing. By the fifteenth century, vernacular poets like John Lydgate and the Oxford chancellor, priest, and physician Gilbert Kymer wrote regimens of health that would allow the educated person to regulate his own lifestyle better to appreciate the nature of the good life. The object of Kymer's regimen, of course, was his patron, the aspiring humanist and book collector Humfrey, duke of Gloucester,[1] whose appetite for women, rather than for food, seems to have worried his physician.

The irony of a physician like Kymer adopting an intellectual stance implying Humfrey ought to be his own physician is obvious enough. But if one considers Gilbert Kymer as the duke's teacher more than his doctor, then Kymer's attitude to his patron becomes clearer. The model for Kymer's regimen was the *Secretum secretorum,* purported to be Aristotle's letters to his student Alexander the Great. It was a model flattering both to Dr. Kymer and to Duke Humfrey. Some of Aristotle's advice was medical, but only in that the king was taught to observe a healthful regimen. Other advice concerned how to choose a good servant, and assorted matters of household management.

Learning how to live well by reading the works of the ancients and maintaining a healthful regimen to preserve vigor into a ripe old age are qualities we associate more with humanism and less with the scholastic medicine taught at English universities, although the distinction between scholastic and humanistic approaches to learning are never clearly observed.[2] Openness, simplicity, practical advice, and writing in the vernacular are also generally humanistic qualities, especially in humanism's earlier forms.[3]

Humanist devotion to openness and simplicity as manifested by writing in the vernacular and by reverence for the writings of the ancient Romans had to a certain extent been present in England since the time of the Anglo-Saxons, who produced translations of late-antique Latin medical texts. The Norman Conquest in 1066 brought a new language of openness—French—but it was a foreign tongue, and by the last quarter of the fourteenth century, native pride in English again became apparent.[4]

One of the first medical texts manifesting this resurgence of medicine in English was the uroscopy of Henry Daniel, written about 1379.[5] Daniel, a Dominican friar, compiled his book on urines in English[6] from a number of Latin sources out of charitable motives because "the more openly taught something is, the more people will take it seriously."[7] English for Daniel, and for other vernacular translators, was not only a tool for teaching and openness but also a rhetorical aid to persuade the reader of the usefulness of this type of medicine.[8]

These medical translations did not arise in a vacuum but were in fact part of a larger movement toward vernacular writing that strengthened in England during the second half of the fourteenth century.[9] Dominicans and Franciscans—Italian orders of friars—were advocates of humanistic ideas about the use of the vernacular for teaching and writing at English universities.[10] The Wycliffite movement, which produced an English translation of the Bible so that more people could see for themselves what Scrip-

ture said, is of course the most famous example of this humanistic/vernac-
ular movement, one that was brutally suppressed by church authorities.[11]

In England, early medical humanism reveals itself most clearly not in
any physician but in medieval England's greatest vernacular poet, Geoffrey
Chaucer (d. 1400). Like learned medicine, Chaucer's humanism seems to
have been imported from Italy and France, whice he visited on diplomatic
missions a number of times in the 1370s. He certainly visited Florence and
became familiar with the Italian language there, as well as with the works
of Boccaccio and Petrarch—and perhaps even the poets themselves.[12]

Petrarch (d. 1374) about 1350 had written his *Invectiva contra medicum*
(Invective against physicians), directed at the multitude of doctors attending Pope Clement VI at Avignon in France. It is a defense of the true
rhetoric of the poet against the false rhetoric of the multitude of physicians
who "belch many things against the poets with that rash, sluggish, vicious
and medicine-smeared tongue."[13] Chaucer's writings display no direct familiarity with the *Invectiva*, but its sentiments against the many discordant
voices of the pope's physicians, obscure and always in disagreement, certainly are present in Chaucer's works.

Chaucer's medical humanism did not exist apart from widespread ideas
about health and disease shared by others of his time. For instance, Chaucer shared with his learned contemporaries certain notions about the
way the body functioned: through the heat of digestion, the body "cooked"
its food, transforming what one ate and drank into the four humors. These
humors (blood, choler, phlegm, and melancholy) nourished the bodily
parts—organs, bones, muscles—which in turn digested this nourishment
according to each one's needs. The superfluities of this digestion were
excreted by the body in the form of urine, feces, menstrual or hemor-
rhoidal blood, flatulence, and sweat. Medical practitioners examined these
superfluities to learn about what was going on inside the body. Learned
medicine is thus called dietetic medicine, from its notion that the central
physiological process was eating and digestion, followed by the purgation
of superfluities.[14]

The state of the body, of course, was ruled by more than just its food.
Dietetic medicine encompassed "diet" in the classical sense of *diaeta*—
one's entire regimen or mode of living. Seen from this point of view, the
way in which the body worked—its physiology—was ruled by several factors.
These were conveniently distilled from the writings of Galen by Islamic
commentators into the so-called nonnaturals: factors outside the body that
affected its well-being. Usually there were six nonnaturals: food, drink, and
fasting; sleep and wakefulness; air; exercise and rest; excretion and retention; and the emotions. Some lists include sexual intercourse and absti-
nence. Moderation of these nonnaturals led to health; unruliness led to
disease. The learned physician, in theory, knew how to teach his patient

the proper regimen or diet yielding good health.[15] Important for understanding Chaucer's medical ideas is to remember that the emotions (or
passions of the soul) had an important effect on the body's well-being.

Chaucer was a respected poet and royal courtier, of course, not a medical
doctor; in fact, his writings give every indication that he shared with Petrarch the deepest contempt for anyone who took money for learned advice, especially physicians.[16] Instead, Chaucer used his medical learning in
an allusive sense, to deepen audience understanding of character and situation. Moreover, like the physician who examined his patients' urine to
discover what went on inside, Chaucer examined the nature of his characters' superfluities and their modes of life to show what sort of persons they
were inside.

Chaucer's most complex usage of medical language and allusion is his
Nun's Priest's Tale, one of the *Canterbury Tales.* It reveals Chaucer's opposi-
tion to medical advice because such concerns lead to folly and vanity. In
this beast epic set in a barnyard, the poet contrasted two types of women.
First, he presented the virtuous, moderate, modest widow, who as a farmer
lived close to nature—"Repleccioun ne made hire nevere sik;/ Attempree
diete was al hir phisik,/ And exercise, and hertes suffisaunce"[17]—whose
"housbondrie" gave her the sort of autonomy admired by the humanistically minded. This paragon was contrasted with the romantically titled
"faire damoysele Pertelote," favorite wife to the gorgeous rooster Chauntecleer, who listened to her husband relate his terrifying dream about
being carried off by a fox and advised all sorts of laxatives to purge the
offending humors causing his nightmare.

A dandy surrounded by women—the human widow and her daughters,
and the "sevene hennes . . . Whiche were his sustres and his paramours"[18]—
the proud rooster chose to follow the wrong example. Everything about
Chauntecleer was excessive: his vanity, his sexuality, his speech, and, most
to the point, his devotion to materialistic explanations of dreams. The
cock's dream was not caused by bad digestion, as Pertelote advised, but
rather was a warning from God, a warning the dreamer was too vain and
dependent on his wife to heed.

Chaucer's lesson in this tale is more than that "Wommannes conseil
broghte us first to wo;"[19] it is about bad and good advice.[20] The individual
knows in his or her heart how best to lead the good life. So did the frugal,
independent widow. Resort to "experts"—and Chaucer delighted to use
medical experts as his bad example—appealed only to vanity and led one
astray. Chauntecleer's problem was moral, not physical. As a result, he very
nearly became part of the fox's diet himself when his dream came true.[21]

Chaucer assumed in his *Nun's Priest's Tale* that moderation in diet and in
moral conduct would lead to happiness and long life. The goatlike Pardoner, another Canterbury pilgrim, who boasted he sold healing relics to

the foolish and desperate, claimed "For though myself be a ful vicious man,/ A moral tale yet I yow telle kan."[22] But his nightmarish story of poisoning, plague, and "superfluytee abhomynable" is anything but moral, in spite of his concluding appeal to "Crist, that is oure soules leche." Similarly, the suspiciously "sangwyn-clad" pilgrim, the Doctour of Phisik, whose pitiful tale of Roman virtue caused the credulous Host to deem the teller "lyk a prelat," was anxious to appear the picture of moderation. Chaucer would have none of it, however: "He kepte that he wan in pestilence./ For gold in phisik is a cordial,/ Therefore he lovede gold in special."[23]

This is not gentle satire. Petrarch was more direct, but Chaucer was no less vicious about medical practitioners, religious or university-educated. The Pardoner and the Doctor were false healers and hypocrites whose appearance betrayed them.[24] The excesses of other pilgrims were similarly, but less fully, revealed by clever use of medical language to suggest what went on inside. The drunken Cook, who made "blankmanger" (white pudding) with the best of them, had a pus-weeping ulcer on his leg. Similarly, the lecherous and drunken Summoner was revealed by his pimply-red face: "Ther nas quyk-silver, lytarge, ne brymstoon,/ Boras, ceruce, ne oille of tartre noon;/ Ne oynement that wolde clense and byte,/ That hym myghte helpen of his whelkes white."[25]

The intimate link between conduct or mode of life and bodily health is much more subtly realized in writings apart from the *Canterbury Tales*. In *Troilus and Criseyde*, Chaucer's epic of the Trojan War, Troilus followed bad advice for his lovesickness and died: a better mentor than his friend Pandarus (from whom we get the word "panderer") would have turned his mind to higher things.[26] Chaucer's favorite nonnatural, sleep, which sends dreams, cured the poet of his melancholy in *The Book of the Duchess*. But perhaps Chaucer's strongest statement on the best way to health was, as with Pliny and Roger Bacon, not to care for material medicines at all. In Chaucer's *Boece*, his translation of the *Consolation of Philosophy* of the Roman philosopher Boethius (executed ca. 524), the narrator, in prison, is encouraged by Lady Philosophy to turn his eyes to the stars, no longer obscured by the clouds and shifting winds. " 'But tyme is now,' " quod sche, 'of medicyne more than of compleynte. . . . Art nat thou he, . . . that whilom, norissched with my melk and fostred with myne metes, were escaped and comyn to courage of a parfit man?' "[27] The narrator continued, "the cloudes of sorowe dissolved and doon awey, I took hevene, and resceyved mynde to knowe the face of my fisycien; so that I sette myne eien on hir and fastned my lookynge. I byholde my noryce [nurse], Philosophie."[28]

Chaucer's beliefs about physiology seem to have been those of the Stoic philosopher and not the physician. The sorrows and ills of this world are only transitory. They can best be endured by practicing dietary and economic moderation. The eternal world, as represented by the stars, is the proper object of the educated person's interest, and estrangement from it the only real disease. For Chaucer then, bodily medicine was, as for Pliny, part of household economy and not philosophy. A Stoic attitude to ills and a moderate lifestyle would lead to well-being, and autonomy, not dependence, would give peace of mind. Chaucer believed that a moderate, economic lifestyle and Stoicism in the face of bodily suffering would prevent illness, including mental distress. The autonomy that economic and intellectual independence brought could leave little place for the medical practitioner, except perhaps as a teacher.[29]

The pressing problems of famine, epidemic disease, and social dislocation among the poor made resort to medical practitioners nearly impossible. When historians remark that there was little in medieval England that medicine actually could do for sick people, what they really mean is that medieval doctors had little in common with modern scientific practitioners. A very important point that is often forgotten applies to care for people living on the margins of society. There was quite a lot that medieval society could do for the hungry, the homeless, the crippled, the unwed mother, the aged, and the orphaned. Society could offer them food, shelter, and protection, which could make a difference between life and death for the needy. The mechanism for offering this sort of care in medieval England was Christian charity, more often than not through hospitals.

The medieval hospital had more in common with its linguistic cousins "hotel," "hospice," and "hospitality" than it did with the modern scientific hospital. Martha Carlin, in her survey of medieval English hospitals, found virtually no evidence of medical care offered by physicians and surgeons. Instead, she found that "treatment most likely to have been available to the sick in hospitals was bed rest, warmth, cleanliness, and an adequate diet."[30] These institutions, funded almost exclusively by charity, served lepers, the needy, the sick poor, the poor traveler, the unwed mother, and, very occasionally, the plague victim.[31] Some hospitals were devoted to the elderly[32] or to the insane.[33] Typically, these institutions were managed on a monastic model, with a strict regimen of diet and prayer, especially prayer for the soul of the institution's benefactor.[34]

The first hospitals in Britain were established by the Roman armies along Continental models. One, built in Perthshire at the end of the first century A.D., could hold more than 250 inmates.[35] After the departure of the Roman invaders, there is no firm evidence of hospitals as independent institutions until the Norman invasion.[36] By the middle of the twelfth century almost seventy such institutions were known to exist; there were nearly five hundred fifty by the early fourteenth century.[37] An early motivation for their foundation was the desire by monastic institutions to provide charity to travelers and the sick poor away from the places where the monks and nuns were housed, so as to prevent too much worldly involvement.[38] Another strong motivation was to house lepers away from cities and monastic houses.[39] Nearly all care was provided by women nurses, with men providing religious supervision.[40]

Hospitals varied enormously in the number of inmates admitted, from fewer than a dozen to nearly two hundred. Continental models figured importantly on a few occasions in the late Middle Ages. London's Savoy, funded by Henry VII, was built on the model of Santa Maria Nuova in Florence, with cubicles for the patients placed in a cruciform church so that they could observe services from their beds.[41] Several crusading orders founded hospitals in England—Knights Templars, Hospitallers, Lazarites of Jerusalem, and Trinitarians, concerned mainly with the care of foreign travelers and lepers. Their numbers were not great—Orme and Webster found only sixty such institutions out of about five hundred in the thirteenth century. Local conditions, they note, dictated the nature of the English hospital much more than foreign influence.[42]

The care offered to medieval English society's most needy no doubt made the difference between life and death for many. Famine and pestilence were everyday facts of life for medieval people, and they affected the poor most of all.[43] It is important to remember that the main purpose of hospital care was not to save lives but to allow the pious to exercise Christian charity through healing.[44] The power of Christ and the saints to heal the sick as a manifestation of divine power was widely believed in by every level of medieval English society. Such faith is not widespread today; we tend to think of "spiritual healing" as a last resort when science fails rather than as the preferred among many alternatives. What is more, as Ronald C. Finucane has insightfully pointed out, historians have shrunk from the historical study of healing miracles: "since most historians do not believe in miracles, they have seen little reason to examine the evidence."[45]

Throughout the medieval period in England there were records of pilgrimages to the shrines of saints for healing. Chaucer's *Canterbury Tales* chronicled the stories told along such a journey to the shrine of St. Thomas Becket at Canterbury, "the hooly blisful martir forto seke,/That hem hath holpen whan that they were seeke."[46] Men and women from all levels of society participated in Chaucer's imaginary pilgrimage, making it a fair reflection of the variety of people who actually sought out religious healing in medieval England.[47]

The shrines of various saints were and are filled with the relics, especially bones, hair, and other bodily fragments, of the holy person.[48] These relics were certainly "symbolic" of the departed martyr, but they were more than that. Like the bread and wine of the Eucharist, the relics of the saint actually were the physical presence of the departed one, in some senses still a person.[49] With a saint as recently martyred as Becket (d. 1170), the real presence of the holy one was very near indeed. The boundary between the living and the dead was not absolute, even after centuries had passed.

The popularity of religious healing, which dates from ancient times, seems, like learned medicine, not to have been impaired in the least by its lack of helpful effect according to modern scientific standards. This enduring attraction may be explained in part by a lack of alternatives. But a partial explanation must also lie in the way medieval English people viewed the boundary between life and death in their own bodies, not just in those of saints. Northern Europeans, especially, tended to see the postmortem dissolution of the link between body and spirit as a gradual one, typically taking a year. During this time, the body decomposed bit by bit, but retained what Katharine Park has called its "selfhood."[50] Beyond that, the boundary between the living and the dead was further obscured by the difficulty medieval people had in determining whether life had actually left a body irretrievably, in the modern sense. One chronicler remarked that revival of the dead after a couple of days was not unusual in England, but that after seven days it was very surprising.[51]

Modern people know much more about the boundaries between physical life and death than did medieval English people; moreover, the likelihood for recovery from a fatal-seeming illness is much easier for scientific physicians to judge than it was for people in prescientific cultures. What might seem a miraculous recovery in the Middle Ages, in short, might be entirely mundane and predictable to the scientific physician. The difficulty prescientific cultures had in predicting the outcome of disease and in judging whether a person would revive are important to understanding why miraculous cures were reported so frequently and thus hoped for fervently.

We know now that the hopes of some medieval English people for medicine without doctors did not really catch on. Medical technology has made unbelievable progress and only a fool would wish it away. But then as now, all lives must come to an end. The human need for a wise and kindly adviser like Gilbert Eagle, who had the learned judgment to determine that death was near and the courage to let the sufferer know it, is with us still. Medieval English medicine may have been a patchwork of foreign imports—texts, institutions, and people—but it also left us with an ideal: the physician as priest and counselor.

Abbreviations Used in Notes

BRUC   Emden, A. B. *A Biographical Register of the University of Cambridge to 1500.*
        Cambridge: Cambridge University Press, 1963.

BRUO   Emden, A. B. *A Biographical Register of the University of Oxford to 1500.* 3
        vols. Oxford: Clarendon Press, 1957–59.

MPME   Talbot, C. H., and E. A. Hammond. *The Medical Practitioners in Medieval
        England: A Biographical Register.* London: Wellcome Historical Medical
        Library, 1965.

MPME/S Getz, Faye. "Medical Practitioners in Medieval England." *Social History of
        Medicine* 3 (1990): 245–83.

TK   Thorndike, Lynn, and Pearl Kibre. *A Catalogue of Incipits of Mediaeval Sci
        entific Writings in Latin.* London: Mediaeval Academy of America, 1963.

Preface

1. Claude Lévi-Strauss, "The Sorcerer and His Magic," in *Structural Anthropology,* trans. Claire Jacobson and Brooke Grundfest Schoepf (New York: Basic Books, 1963), pp. 167–85.

2. Ibid., p. 180.

Chapter I
The Variety of Medical Practitioners
in Medieval England

1. *Radulphi de Coggeshall Chronicon Anglicanum,* ed. Joseph Stevenson, Rolls Series 66 (London: Longman, 1875), pp. 156–59. On Gilbert and his relationship to Hubert and Henry le Afaitie (Lafaitie), see C. H. Talbot and E. A. Hammond, *The Medical Practitioners in Medieval England: A Biographical Register* (London: Wellcome Historical Medical Library, 1965), pp. 58–60; hereafter *MPME.* The identity of Gilbertus Anglicus with Gillbertus del Egle was demonstrated by Ernest Wickersheimer in his *Dictionnaire biographique des médecins en France au moyen âge* (Paris: Librairie E. Droz, 1936), pp. 191–92.

2. *Profession, Vocation, and Culture in Later Medieval England: Essays Dedicated to the Memory of A. R. Myers,* ed. Cecil Clough (Liverpool: Liverpool University Press, 1982).

3. Margaret Pelling and Charles Webster, "Medical Practitioners," in *Health, Medicine, and Mortality in the Sixteenth Century,* ed. Charles Webster (Cambridge: Cambridge University Press, 1979), pp. 165–235; Margaret Pelling, "Occupational Diversity: Barbersurgeons and the Trades of Norwich, 1550–1640," *Bulletin of the History of Medicine* 56 (1982): 484–511.

4. Margaret Pelling, "Medical Practice in Early Modern England: Trade or Profession?" in *The Professions in Early Modern England,* ed. W. Prest (London: Croom Helm, 1987), pp. 90–128.

5. Harold J. Cook, *The Decline of the Old Medical Regime in Stuart London* (Ithaca, N.Y.: Cornell University Press, 1986), esp. "The Medical Marketplace of London," pp. 28–69.

6. The development of medicine as a profession on the European continent, especially northern Italy, contrasts sharply with England. For medieval views on the medical profession in general, see Nancy G. Siraisi, *Medieval and Early Renaissance Medicine: An Introduction to Knowledge and Practice* (Chicago: University of Chicago Press, 1990), pp. 17–23.

7. My findings for England may be contrasted with those of Danielle Jacquart in *Le milieu médical en France du XIIe au XVe siècle, en annexe 2e supplément au Dictionnaire d'Ernest Wickersheimer* (Geneva: Librairie Droz, 1981), pp. 27–55. Jacquart finds categories of practitioners for France that seem more rigid and developed than were those in England.

8. My findings for medieval England may be compared with those of Michael R. McVaugh for the Crown of Aragon in the first half of the fourteenth century; *Medicine before the Plague: Practitioners and Their Patients in the Crown of Aragon, 1285–1345* (Cambridge: Cambridge University Press, 1993), see esp. pp. 241–45. McVaugh's close study of a large amount of data over a short time period enabled him to document a rapidly growing community of practitioners, with increasingly specialized and standardized expertise, whose development was spurred on by lay patronage and demand.

9. In general, see Carole Rawcliffe, "Women and Medicine: Conflicting Attitudes" and "Women and Medicine: The Midwife and the Nurse," in *Medicine and Society in Later Medieval England* (Stroud: Alan Sutton, 1995), pp. 170–93, 194–215.

10. For venality among the more elite English medical practitioners, see Carole Rawcliffe, "The Profits of Practice: The Wealth and Status of Medical Men in Later Medieval England," *Social History of Medicine* 1 (1988): 61–78; also, more sympathetically, E. A. Hammond, "Incomes of Medieval English Doctors," *Journal of the History of Medicine* 15 (1960): 154–69.

11. A summary of the ideal motives of the clerical practitioner is John A. Alford, "Medicine in the Middle Ages: The Theory of a Profession," *Centennial Review* 23 (1979): 377–96. For medical writing as a charitable activity, see Faye Marie Getz, "Charity, Translation, and the Language of Medical Learning in Medieval England," *Bulletin of the History of Medicine* 64 (1990): 1–17.

12. *MPME*, p. 106.

13. Stuart Jenks, "Medizinische Fachkräfte in England zur Zeit Heinrichs VI (1428/29–1460/61)," *Sudhoffs Archiv* 69 (1985): 222–24; *MPME*, p. 280; Faye Marie Getz, "Medical Practitioners in Medieval England," *Social History of Medicine* 3 (1990): 274. The last is a supplement to *MPME*, hereafter cited as *MPME/S*.

14. London, Corporation of London Records Office, Miscellaneous Roll CC, membrane 17 dorse; John was attached for trespass on 29 August 1320; *MPME*, p. 137.

15. Edward J. Kealey, *Medieval Medicus: A Social History of Anglo-Norman Medicine* (Baltimore, Md.: The Johns Hopkins University Press, 1981), p. 86; *MPME/S*, p. 280.

16. *MPME*, pp. 48–49. The Italian Pancio da Controne was also involved with the London wool trade during the first half of the fourteenth century; *MPME*, pp. 234–37; *MPME/S*, p. 271.

17. *MPME*, p. 82.

18. *MPME*, p. 378. Simon de Plaghe, a London physician, received a brewery from vintner John Chaucer, the father of the poet Geoffrey, in 1354; *MPME*, p. 324; *MPME/S*, p. 277. For the complex history of this property, see *Chaucer Life-Records*, ed. Martin M. Crow and Clair C. Olson from materials compiled by John M. Manly and Edith Rickert, with the assistance of Lilian J. Redstone and others (London: Oxford University Press, 1966), pp. 5–7. This particular transaction is not mentioned in the *Life-Records*.

19. James K. Mustain, "A Rural Medical Practitioner in Fifteenth-Century England," *Bulletin of the History of Medicine* 46 (1972): 469–76.

20. Crophill's poem is in his own notebook, now British Library, Harley MS 1735, and is printed by Rossell Hope Robbins in "John Crophill's Ale-Pots," *Review of English Studies*, n.s., 20, no. 78 (1969): 182–89.

21. Robbins, "Alepots," p. 188. Crophill's work in Harley MS 1735 is the subject of a doctoral dissertation at the Centre for Medieval Studies, University of Toronto, by Lois J. Ayoub.

22. *MPME*, p. 123; corrected by S. J. Lang, "John Bradmore and His Book *Philomena*," *Social History of Medicine* 5 (1992): 121–30.

23. G. E. Trease and J. H. Hodson, "The Inventory of John Hexham, A Fifteenth-Century Apothecary," *Medical History* 9 (1965): 76–81.

24. "Leech" was a common English word for any type of medical practitioner, including the surgeon. It was in use in Old English, the language of the Anglo-Saxons. See *Oxford English Dictionary*, s.v. "leech," and *Middle English Dictionary* (Ann Arbor: University of Michigan Press, 1956–   ), s.v. "leche." The term is the usual translation for Latin "medicus." "Leech" is found in the feminine gender; *MPME*, p. 211: "Matilda," *la leche*.

25. This is the Anglo-Norman equivalent of "leech." Anglo-Norman is the language of the French invaders of England, especially during the twelfth and thirteenth centuries. See "mire" and "mirie" in *Anglo-Norman Dictionary*, ed. Louise W. Stone and William Rothwell (London: The Modern Humanities Research Association, 1985). Also, compare with usage in France: Jacquart, in *Le milieu médical*, found the word could denote either a physician or a surgeon (pp. 37–39). For *medicus* and *le mire*, see *MPME*, "Alan of Wallingford," p. 11.

26. Medic; a Latin term for any sort of medical practitioner. It is found in the feminine gender; *MPME/S*, p. 277: "Solicita," *medica*. See also *Promptorium Parvulorum Sive Clericorum*, ed. Albertus Way (Camden Society, 1843), an English-Latin translation dictionary compiled about 1440: "leche, mann or woman. Medicus, medica" (p. 291).

27. Surgeon; medieval spellings for this and other words could vary enormously. Like "leech," the various words for surgeon could be used in a metaphorical sense, especially with reference to spiritual healing. See *Middle English Dictionary*, s.v. "cirurgien." Surgeon is found in the feminine gender; *MPME*, p. 200: "Katherine," *la surgiene*.

28. Physician; the word was more limited in usage than "leech" or "surgeon." Scholarly documents employ the word to imply textual learning and a knowledge of science or theory. In contrast to "leech" and "surgeon," the term is not often used metaphorically, and is usually distinguished from the designation of "surgeon." See *Middle*

English Dictionary, s.vv. "phisike" and "phisicien." I have never encountered *physicus* in the feminine gender. The subtleties involved in understanding the word are explored in Jerome J. Bylebyl, "The Medical Meaning of *Physica*," *Osiris*, 2d ser., 6 (1990): 16–41.

29. From Greek *archiatros*, or head physician. In Anglo-Latin sources, the infrequent usages seem to imply both a spiritual and medical healing context; *Dictionary of Medieval Latin from British Sources*, prepared by R. E. Latham (London: Oxford University Press for the British Academy, 1975), s.v. "archiater."

30. *Middle English Dictionary*, s.v. "maister."

31. *MPME*, pp. 217, 231.

32. Ibid., p. 291.

33. *MPME/S*, pp. 262, 263, 275.

34. For example, "Master Fisicus," *MPME*, p. 211, and "Master Medicus," *MPME*, p. 215.

35. Halyday was a member first of the Fellowship of Barbers (1471), then of the Surgeons' Company (1489), and then of the Barber-Surgeons (1497). Ibid., p. 296.

36. Child: *MPME*, p. 132, *MPME/S*, p. 264; Dalton: *MPME*, p. 140, *MPME/S*, p. 265.

37. *MPME/S*, pp. 257, 263.

38. Ibid., p. 269.

39. *MPME*, pp. 209–10.

40. Martha Carlin, *Medieval Southwark* (London: The Hambledon Press, 1996), pp. 174–77; Judith M. Bennett, "Medieval Women, Modern Woman: Across the Great Divide," in *Culture and History, 1350–1600: Essays on English Communities, Identities and Writing*, ed. David Aers (London: Harvester Wheatsheaf, 1992), p. 156.

41. Leslie G. Matthews, *The Royal Apothecaries* (London: Wellcome Historical Medical Library, 1967), p. 9.

42. *MPME*, p. 237; *MPME/S*, p. 271. For a fuller account of Peter's life, and of other apothecaries like him, see Matthews, *The Royal Apothecaries*, pp. 1–60.

43. The names of women medical practitioners sometimes have been edited from present-day historical writing. See *MPME/S*, p. 248 n. 16.

44. *MPME*, p. 209. See also Matilda, *la leche*, of Wallingford, Berkshire, who in 1232 was assessed 20d. in taxes, more than any other woman in town; *MPME*, p. 211.

45. E. A. Hammond, "Physicians in Medieval English Religious Houses," *Bulletin of the History of Medicine* 32 (1958): 105–20.

46. Eileen Power, *Medieval English Nunneries, c. 1275–1535* (Cambridge: Cambridge University Press, 1922), p. 134. There is also evidence from thirteenth-century France; see p. 649.

47. *MPME/S*, pp. 257, 263.

48. Ibid., p. 263.

49. *MPME*, p. 193. Also holding this title was Robert of St. Albans, ca. 1320–23, who received the same annual stipend; *MPME*, p. 299. An overview of this rich source is E. A. Hammond, "The Westminster Abbey Infirmarers' Rolls as a Source of Medical History," *Bulletin of the History of Medicine* 39 (1965): 261–76.

50. *MPME*, p. 128.

51. Ibid., p. 124.

52. Ibid., p. 209.

53. *MPME*/S, p. 256: "Anonymous. Medicus."

54. *MPME*, p. 331.

55. *MPME*, p. 200; also see *MPME*, pp. 227–28, for Cecilia, *la leche*, who owned a tenement in Oxford ca. 1350, which passed to Robert, *le leche*, and then to his son Nicholas, *le leche*.

56. *MPME*/S, pp. 263, 269, 277; in more detail in Edward J. Kealey, "England's Earliest Women Doctors," *Journal of the History of Medicine* 40 (1985): 473–77.

57. Heather Swanson, "The Illusion of Economic Structure: Craft Guilds in Late Medieval English Towns," *Past and Present* no. 121 (1988): 34–35.

58. *MPME*, pp. 241, 353.

59. *MPME*/S, pp. 266, 277. See also the careers of London surgeons John Bradmore and Nicholas Bradmore, in all likelihood brothers, who flourished around the end of the fourteenth and beginning of the fifteenth centuries; *MPME*, pp. 123, 218; *MPME*/S, pp. 264, 270. Also *The Cutting Edge: Early History of the Surgeons of London*, ed. R. Theodore Beck (London: Lund Humphries, 1974), p. 161; and Lang, "John Bradmore."

60. *MPME*, p. 108.

61. On medieval London guilds in general, see Elspeth M. Veale, "Craftsmen and the Economy of London in the Fourteenth Century," in *Studies in London History Presented to Philip Edmund Jones*, ed. A. E. J. Hollaender and William Kellaway (London: Hodder and Stoughton, 1969), pp. 133–51.

62. English material on surgical apprenticeship is found in Vern L. Bullough, "Training of the Nonuniversity-Educated Medical Practitioners in the Later Middle Ages," *Journal of the History of Medicine* 14 (1959): 446–58.

63. *MPME*, p. 219.

64. *MPME*, pp. 74–75; *MPME*/S, p. 261.

65. *MPME*, pp. 195, 292–93.

66. Ibid., p. 338.

67. Ibid., pp. 293, 352.

68. John Hobbes's will is printed in *Cutting Edge*, pp. 161–62; also see *MPME*, p. 156, and *MPME*/S, p. 266. For the elder John Dagvyle, see *MPME*, p. 139, and *MPME*/S, p. 265.

69. *MPME*, p. 139.

70. *Cutting Edge*, p. 161.

71. *MPME*, p. 140.

72. *MPME*, pp. 401–2; *MPME*/S, p. 282.

73. *Bede's Ecclesiastical History of the English People*, ed. Bertram Colgrave and R. A. B. Mynors (Oxford: Clarendon Press, 1969), pp. 456–59 (bk. 5, chap. 2).

74. *Bede's History*, pp. 458–63 (bk. 5, chap. 3).

75. *MPME*, pp. 259–60; Frank Barlow, *The English Church, 1066–1154* (New York: Longman, 1979), p. 260 n.

76. The cellarer was in charge of food and other provisions for the abbey and was second only to the abbot. The Benedictine rule instructs that the cellarer dispense food like a father (*sicut pater*); *The Rule of St. Benedict: In Latin and English with Notes*, ed. Timothy Fry et al. (Collegeville, Minn.: The Liturgical Press, 1981), pp. 226–27 (chap. 31).

77. *MPME*, pp. 45–46; Kealey, *Medicus*, pp. 65–70.

78. "Lucas quoque medicus, cuius laus per omnes Ecclesias . . . est" ("Vita S. Aldhelmi Faricio Auctore," in *Patrologiae Cursus Completus: Series Latina*, vol. 89 [Paris: J.-P. Migne, 1850], col. 65).

79. *Chronicon monasterii de Abingdon*, ed. Joseph Stevenson, Rolls Series vol. 2, pt. 2 (London: Longman, 1858), p. 50.

80. Kealey, *Medicus*, p. 67.

81. "Probatissimus officio medicus, adeo ut ejus solius antidotum confectionibus rex ipse se crederet saepe medendum" (*Chronicon Abingdon*, p. 44). The use of *antidotum* here may indicate that Faritius alone was trusted to prepare antidotes to poison for the king.

82. Contra mortem nulla est medicina (*Chronicon Abingdon*, p. 55; Kealey, *Medicus*, p. 67). Cf. *Seneca ad Lucilium Epistulae Morales*, trans. Richard M. Gummere, vol. 3, Loeb Classical Library (New York: Putnam's Sons, 1925), letter 94: "Ne medicina quidem morbos insanabiles vincit" (pp. 26–27).

83. *Chronicon Abingdon*, p. 289.

84. Kealey, *Medicus*, p. 68.

85. See, for example, the "informal" medical learning of the Italian Grimbald, who attended Queen Matilda along with Faritius, and that of the monastic chronicler William of Malmesbury, *MPME*, p. 67; Kealey, *Medicus*, p. 66.

86. "Fuit enim sicut non usquequaque despicabilis eloquentiae, ita in his duntaxat, propter ignorantiam linguae, incuriosae scientiae, utpote sub Tusco natus aere" (*Willelmi Malmesbiriensis monachi de gestis pontificum anglorum*, ed. N. E. S. A. Hamilton, Rolls Series 52 [1870; reprint, Nendeln: Kraus, 1965], pp. 330–31). Malmesbury quoted the poetry of Peter, monk of Malmesbury, on Faritius: "Omnibus imbutus quas monstrat phisica leges,/Ipsos demeruit medicandi munere reges./Reges et proceres subici parere videres,/Illius ad nutum credentes vivere tutum" (*De gestis pontificum*, pp. 192–93).

87. Kealey, *Medicus*, pp. 68–69.

88. "Eo tempore obiit Anselmus archiepiscopus; tunc electus est Faricius ad archiepiscopatum, sed episcopus Lincolniensis et episcopus Salesburiensis obstiterunt, dicentes non debere archiepiscopum urinas mulierum inspicere" (*Chronicon Abingdon*, p. 287).

89. "Si Longobardus ille fuerit archiepiscopus, rursus lites, rursus discidia. . . . Satis superque alienae gentis homines fuisse archiepiscopos. Abundare patriae linguae viros" (William of Malmesbury, *De gestis pontificum*, p. 126). "Longobardus" here simply means "Italian."

90. *MPME*, pp. 130–31.

91. In Grammatica Priscianus, in metrico Ovidius, in Physica censeri potuit Galienus (*Gesta Abbatum Monasterii Sancti Albani, a Thoma Walsingham*, ed. Henry Thomas Riley, vol. 1, A.D. *793–1290*. Rolls Series 28, vol. 1, pt. 4, [London: Longman, 1867], p. 217). The Rolls Series presents Thomas Walsingham's later version of Matthew Paris's original *Gesta abbatum: Chronicles of Matthew Paris: Monastic Life in the Thirteenth Century*, ed., trans., and with an introduction by Richard Vaughn (New York: St. Martin's Press, 1984), p. 10. Vaughn's translation of Matthew's accolade of John of Cella is found on p. 14.

92. *MPME*, pp. 130–31.
93.

In crastino autem diligenter consideravit urinam suam, quidnam portenderit; erat enim, ut praedictum est, physicus praeelectus, et judex urinarum incomparabilis. Et cum intuitus est diligenter, nec posset ad placitum subtilia et secreta, quae novit, mortis indicia intueri, quia caligaverat in magna parte suorum acies oculorum, dixit Magistro Willelmo physico, monacho nostro, (qui postea in priorem Wygorniae promotus est);—"Quid tu vides hic et hic, frater?" At ipse quae vidit indicavit. At Abbas,— "Eya, Deo gratias. Adhuc concessit mihi Deus, ad poenitentiam, spatium triduanum; sed post tres dies dissolvar." Quod qui audierunt, bene crediderunt; quia experientissimus in arte medicinae erat. (*Gesta . . . Walsingham*, p. 246; Paris, *Gesta abbatum* [much less detailed], pp. 29–30)

For William of Bedford, see *MPME*, p. 384.
94. *MPME*, pp. 223–24.
95. Ibid., p. 225.
96. Ibid., p. 224.
97. Virum grandeum et regis medicum qui de medico corporum factus est medicus animarum (*The Chronicle of Melrose: A Complete and Full-Size Facsimile in Collotype*, with an introduction by Alan Orr Anderson and Marjorie Ogilvie Anderson, and an index by William Croft Dickinson [London: Percy Lund Humphries, 1936], p. 88, lines 4–5); *MPME*, p. 225 n. 18.
98. "Ipsum igitur quasi expertum, et scientia multipliciter et morbis commendabilibus insignitum, peritorum consilio rex et regina ad suarum vocaverunt animarum et corporum custodiam et consilium familiare, hos consulentibus et procurantibus Ottone tunc legato et episcopo Carleolensi et aliis secretis regis consiliariis" (*Matthaei Parisiensis, Monachi Sancti Albani, Chronica Majora*, vol. 4, A.D. *1240–1247*, ed. Henry Richards Luard, Rolls Series 57 [London: Longman, 1877], pp. 86–87). Popes and cardinals contemporary with Farnham also employed physicians as chaplains. See, for example, "Remigio" and "Bonaventura" in Agostino Paravicini Bagliani, *Medicina e scienze della natura alla corte dei papi nel duecento* (Spoleto: Centro Italiano di Studi Sull'Alto Medioevo, 1991), p. 23.
99. *MPME*, p. 225.

His igitur et aliis sanctitatis argumentis certificatus episcopus Dunelmensis Nicholaus, quem adeo hydropisis incurabilis undique dilataverat, ictericia decoloraverat, macies attenuaverat et substantialem humiditatem consumpserat, tussis desiccaverat, asma inquietaverat, certa quoque mortis imminentia denigraverat, ut solum sibi superesse sepulchrum videretur, omni humano destitutus et desperatus auxilio, fide plenus confugit ad divinum. Vovit igitur se sepulchrum beati Edmundi Cantuariensis archiepiscopi devote cum honore visitaturum, si sic corporalis convalescentia pateretur. . . . Habuit autem quendam suum ministrum, W. nomine, qui aliquando tonsor beati Edmundi Cantuariensis archiepiscopi et ostiarius extiterat; hic in spiritu comperiens, quod ipsum archipraesulem Deus non immerito sanctorum annumeraret collegio, pilos barbae suae, quam radere solebat, reservaverat, sperans eos in futuro aegris profuturos. Hoc cum episcopo Nicholao jam semivivo, qui tamen memoria viguit, innuit, praecepit ministro memorato, ut pili illi in aqua benedicta sibi darentur ad bibendum; quam cum exhauserat, vomitu sedatus omnis tumor et omnis dolor penitus mitigatus. Et sic brevi plenae restitutus est sanitati." (*Matthaei Parisiensis . . . Chronica Majora*, p. 330)

100. *MPME/S*, p. 265. Like Nicholas of Farnham, John was part of Robert Grosseteste's intellectual circle. John petitioned the pope unsuccessfully in 1307 to have his great predecessor as bishop of Lincoln canonized; Jennifer R. Bray, "Concepts of Sainthood in Fourteenth-Century England," *Bulletin of the John Rylands University Library of Manchester* 66 (1983–84): 49.

101. *MPME*, pp. 92–93; Paravicini Bagliani, *Medicina e scienze della natura*, pp. 262–64. A recipe for lung disease attributed to him is in Gloucester Cathedral manuscript 18; *MPME/S*, p. 262. On the fortunes of other works attributed to him, mostly both alchemical and medical, and written in association with the English Cistercian cardinal John of Toledo, see Paravicini Bagliani, *Medicina e scienze della natura*, pp. 402–5.

102. *MPME*, p. 362; *MPME/S*, p. 279.

103. Johannes Blund, *Tractatus de anima*, ed. D. A. Callus and R. W. Hunt (London: Oxford University Press, 1970). See also Faye Marie Getz, "The Faculty of Medicine before 1500," in *The History of the University of Oxford*, vol. 2, *Late Medieval Oxford*, ed. Jeremy Catto and Ralph Evans (Oxford: Clarendon Press, 1992), pp. 385–86.

104. *Alfred of Sareshel (Alfredus Anglicus), De motu cordis*, ed. Clemens Baeumker, *Beiträge zur Geschichte der Philosophie des Mittelalters* 23 (1923): pts. 1–2. Also Getz, "Faculty of Medicine," pp. 385–86 and *MPME/S*, p. 255.

105. Bartholomaeus Anglicus, *De proprietatibus rerum* (1601; reprint, Frankfurt am Main: Minerva G. M. B. H., 1964). The work was translated into English by John Trevisa and completed in February 1398–99: *On the Properties of Things: John Trevisa's Translation of* Bartholomaeus Anglicus De Proprietatibus Rerum, *A Critical Text*, ed. M. C. Seymour et al., vol. 1 (Oxford: Clarendon Press, 1975), p. xi.

106. Getz, "Faculty of Medicine," pp. 386–87. The medical material covers book 7; *On the Properties of Things*, pp. 342–440.

107. Vern L. Bullough, "Medical Study at Mediaeval Oxford," *Speculum* 36 (1961): 603–5.

108. *MPME*, pp. 58–60; *MPME/S*, p. 259.

109. *MPME*, pp. 270–72; *MPME/S*, p. 274; Paravicini Bagliani, *Medicina e scienze della natura*, pp. 17–20; Wickersheimer, *Dictionnaire biographique*, pp. 695–98.

110. *MPME/S*, p 276.

111. See Getz, "Faculty of Medicine," and Damian Riehl Leader, "Medicine," in *A History of the University of Cambridge*, vol. 1, *The University to 1546* (Cambridge: Cambridge University Press, 1988), pp. 202–10.

112. *MPME*, p. 323; *MPME/S*, p. 277; A. B. Emden, *A Biographical Register of the University of Oxford to 1500* (Oxford: Clarendon Press, 1957–59), 2:945; hereafter *BRUO*. On the manuscripts, see R. A. B. Mynors, *Catalogue of the Manuscripts of Balliol College Oxford* (Oxford: Clarendon Press, 1963), MS 231, pp. 244–47; ascription on fol. 1v; Montague Rhodes James, *A Descriptive Catalogue of the Manuscripts in the Library of Peterhouse* (Cambridge: Cambridge University Press, 1899), MS 140, pp. 166–67: *Johannes Fil. Serapionis de Simplicibus Medicinis Etc.* instructions on fol. 1.

113. *MPME*, pp. 221–22; *MPME*/S, p. 270.

114. *MPME*, p. 335.

115. *MPME*, p. 134; *BRUO*, 3; 2163–64.

116. *MPME*, p. 220.

117. Guy Fitch Lytle, "The Social Origins of Oxford Students in the Late Middle Ages: New College, c. 1380–1510," in *The Universities in the Late Middle Ages*, ed. Jozef IJsewijn and Jacques Paquet (Louvain: Leuven University Press, 1978), pp. 426–54.

118. *MPME*, pp. 203–4; *MPME*/S, p. 269.

119. *MPME*, pp. 96–98; *MPME*/S, p. 262.

120. *MPME*, pp. 115–16; *MPME*/S, p. 263.

121. *MPME*, p. 143; *MPME*/S, p. 265; *BRUO*, 1; 663.

122. *MPME*, pp. 184–85; *MPME*/S, p. 267.

123. *MPME*, p. 60.

Chapter II
Medical Travelers to England and the English
Medical Practitioner Abroad

1. Joe Hillaby, "London: The 13th-Century Jewry Revisited," *Jewish Historical Studies: Transactions of the Jewish Historical Society of England* 32 (1990–92): 135; Gwyn A. Williams, *Medieval London: From Commune to Capital* (London: Athlone Press, 1963), p. 224.

2. Sylvia L. Thrupp, "A Survey of the Alien Population of England in 1440," *Speculum* 32 (1958): 265.

3. V. D. Lipman, *The Jews of Medieval Norwich* (London: Jewish Historical Society of England, 1967), pp. 160–61.

4. Cecil Roth, "Elijah of London: The Most Illustrious English Jew of the Middle Ages," *Transactions of the Jewish Historical Society of England* 15 (1939–45): 40.

5. D. Cohn-Sherbok, "Medieval Jewish Persecution in England: The Canterbury Pogroms in Perspective," *Southern History* 3 (1981): 23–37; R. B. Dobson, "The Jews of Medieval Cambridge," *Jewish Historical Studies: Transactions of the Jewish Historical Society of England* 32 (1990–92): 1–24; Dobson, "The Decline and Expulsion of the Medieval Jews of York," *Jewish Historical Studies: Transactions of the Jewish Historical Society of England* 26 (1974–78): 34–52; Hillaby, "London," pp. 89–158; Hillaby, "A Magnate among the Marchers: Hamo of Hereford, His Family and Clients, 1218–1253," *Jewish Historical Studies: Transactions of the Jewish Historical Society of England* 31 (1988–90): 23–82; Lipman, *Norwich*; Cecil Roth, *The Jews of Medieval Oxford*, Oxford Historical Society, n.s., 9 (Oxford: Clarendon Press, 1951).

6. Kevin T. Streit, "The Expansion of the English Jewish Community in the Reign of King Stephen," *Albion* 25 (1993): 177–92.

7. On popular anti-Semitic fantasies among English Christians, see Gavin I. Langmuir, "The Knight's Tale and Young Hugh of Lincoln," *Speculum* 47 (1972): 459–82; and his "Thomas of Monmouth: Detector of Ritual Murder," *Speculum* 59 (1984): 820–46.

8. T. P. McLaughlin, "The Teaching of the Canonists on Usury (XII, XIII and XIV Centuries)," *Mediaeval Studies* 1 (1939): 81–147.

9. Robin Mundill, "Anglo-Jewry under Edward I: Credit Agents and Their Clients," *Jewish Historical Studies: Transactions of the Jewish Historical Society of England* 31 (1988–90): 1; more generally, John H. Munro, "Bullionism and the Bill of Exchange in England, 1272–1663: A Study in Monetary Management and Popular Prejudice," in *The Dawn of Modern Banking* (New Haven, Conn.: Yale University Press, 1979), pp. 169–239.

10. H. G. Richardson, *The English Jewry under Angevin Kings* (London: Methuen, 1960), pp. 140–42.

11. Dobson, "Cambridge," suggests that the Hospital of St. John, first mentioned in 1204, which stood across the street from the Cambridge Jewry, loaned money from its start in deliberate competition with the Jews (p. 15).

12. Dobson has noted the likelihood that Christian usury preceded the arrival of the Jews in England; "York," p. 41.

13. Robin Mundill, "The Jewish Entries from the Patent Rolls, 1272–1292," *Jewish Historical Studies: Transactions of the Jewish Historical Society of England* 32 (1990–92): 25.

14. Dobson, "Cambridge," pp. 16–17; Hillaby, "London," p. 101.

15. Zefira Entin Rokéah, "Money and the Hangman in Late-13th-Century England: Jews, Christians and Coinage Offences Alleged and Real (Part I)," *Jewish Historical Studies: Transactions of the Jewish Historical Society of England* 31 (1988–90): 98–99.

16. Robert Chazan, *Daggers of Faith: Thirteenth-Century Christian Missionizing and Jewish Response* (Berkeley: University of California Press, 1989), p. 45.

17. R. W. Hunt, "The Disputation of Peter of Cornwall against Symon the Jew," in *Studies in Medieval History Presented to Frederick Maurice Powicke*, ed. R. W. Hunt, W. A. Pantin, and R. W. Southern (Oxford: Clarendon Press, 1948), pp. 143–56, outlines Christian strategies to convert the Jews and to refute their arguments in England during the eleventh and twelfth centuries.

18. Jeremy Cohen, *The Friars and the Jews: The Evolution of Medieval Anti-Judaism* (Ithaca, N.Y.: Cornell University Press, 1982), p. 43.

19. Lipman, *Norwich*, p. 37. For a Continental comparison, see Michael R. McVaugh, "Jewish Practitioners," in *Medicine before the Plague: Practitioners and Their Patients in the Crown of Aragon, 1285–1345* (Cambridge: Cambridge University Press, 1993), pp. 55–64.

20. Robert Chazan, *Medieval Jewry in Northern France: A Political and Social History* (Baltimore, Md.: The Johns Hopkins University Press, 1973), p. 183.

21. Cecil Roth, *A History of the Jews in England*, 3d ed. (Oxford: Clarendon Press, 1964), pp. 132–35.

22. For a general study of Jewish medicine in Europe during the Middle Ages concentrating on southern France, see Joseph Shatzmiller, *Jews, Medicine, and Medieval Society* (Berkeley: University of California Press, 1994).

23. Hillaby, "London," p. 116.

24. Richard W. Emery, in "Jewish Physicians in Medieval Perpignan," *Michael: On the History of the Jews in the Diaspora* 12 (1991); 113–34, found that between about 1250 and 1418 no Jewish physician made a living exclusively through medical practice and that some also loaned money (p. 116).

25. On the *scola Iudeorum*, see Hillaby, "London," p. 100.

26. *MPME/*S, p. 258; Hillaby, "London," pp. 143–46; Roth, "Elijah," pp. 29–62.

27. Hillaby, "London," p. 144; a list of his writings, none medical, are in Roth, "Elijah," pp. 55–57.

28. Roth, "Elijah," p. 37.

29. Ibid., p. 40.

30. Hillaby, "London," p. 145.

31. Isaac Alteras, "Notes généalogiques sur les médecins juifs dans le sud de la France pendant les XIIIe et XIVe siècles," *Le moyen âge* 88 (1982): 29–47.

32. *MPME*, pp. 95, 326; Lipman, *Norwich*, p. 17; *Shetarot: Hebrew Deeds of English Jews before 1290*, ed. M. D. Davis, Publications of the Anglo-Jewish Historical Exhibition 2 (London, 1888), p. 132, no. 52.

33. Roth, *Oxford*, p. 127.

34. Emery suggests that this was the case in Perpignan; "Jewish Physicians," p. 116.

35. Hillaby, "Hamo of Hereford," p. 29.

36. *MPME*, p. 317; Cecil Roth, "The Qualification of Jewish Physicians in the Middle Ages," *Speculum* 28 (1953): 834; *Calendar of the Plea Rolls of the Exchequer of the Jews*, vol. 2, *Edward I, 1273–1275*, ed. J. M. Rigg (Edinburgh: Ballantyne, Hanson and Co., 1910), p. 14.

37. For a survey of the study of the Hebrew language in England among Christians, see Mark Zier, "The Healing Power of the Hebrew Tongue: An Example from Late Thirteenth-Century England," in *Health, Disease and Healing in Medieval Culture*, ed. Sheila Campbell, Bert Hall, and David Klausner (New York: St. Martin's Press, 1992), pp. 103–18.

38. *MPME*, pp. 100–101; Cecil Roth, "Jewish Physicians in Medieval England," *Medical Leaves* 5 (1943): 42–43. "Quidam Judaeus, insignis medicus, qui et artis et modestiae suae gratia Christianis quoque familiaris atque honorabilis fuerat, caedem suorum paulo immoderatius deploravit, et quasi ultionem prophetans, spriantem adhuc furorem instigavit. Quem mox Christiani correptum, ultimam ibidem Judiacae vesaniae victimam fecerunt" (*Chronicles of the Reigns of Stephen, Henry II, and Richard II*, vol. 1, *Containing the First Four Books of the* Historia Rerum Anglicarum *of William of Newburgh*, ed. Richard Howlett, Rolls Series 82 [1884; reprint, Nendeln: Kraus, 1964], p. 310).

39. *MPME*, p. 42. Hillaby, "London," p. 145, suggests that Elijah wanted to leave England in order to avoid molestation by a business rival. Roth, "Elijah," supplies a translation of the letter into English; see also Roth, "Jewish Physicians," p. 45. The original letter is printed with related documents and commentary in Joseph Jacobs, "Une lettre française d'un juif anglais au XIIIe siècle," *Revue des études juives* 18 (1889): 256–61, with the citation on p. 258. The family in question are the descendants by two marriages of Countess Margaret, who ruled Flanders from 1244 to 1279. On the commercial and dynastic contacts of this family with England, see Nellie Kerling, *Commercial Relations of Holland and Zeeland with England from the Late 13th Century to the Close of the Middle Ages* (Leiden: E. J. Brill, 1954), pp. 4–9; also Shatzmiller, *Jews*, p. 66.

40. *MPME/S*, p. 271. A summary of his life and writings is in Edward J. Kealey, *Medieval Medicus: A Social History of Anglo-Norman Medicine* (Baltimore, Md.: The Johns Hopkins University Press, 1981), pp. 75–79. On evidence for Petrus's association with Henry I, see John Tolan, *Petrus Alfonsi and His Medieval Readers* (Gainesville: University Press of Florida, 1993), pp. 10–11. On his alchemical interests, see Alfred Büchler, "A Twelfth-Century Physician's Desk Book: The *Secreta Secretorum* of Petrus Alphonsi

Quondam Moses Sephardi," *Journal of Jewish Studies* 37 (1986): 206–12; also Dorothee Metlitzki, *The Matter of Araby in Medieval England* (New Haven, Conn.: Yale University Press, 1977), pp. 16–26.

41. *MPME*/S, p. 277; Cecil Roth, "The Middle Period of Anglo-Jewish History (1290–1655) Reconsidered," *Jewish Historical Society of England Transactions* 19 (1955–59): 1–2. Samson appears to have come from Mirabeau, which is near the great medical school of Montpellier; Ernest Wickersheimer, *Dictionnaire biographique des médecins en France au Moyen Age* (Paris: Librairie E. Droz, 1936), p. 731; see also A. Weiner, "A Note on Jewish Doctors in England in the Reign of Henry IV," *Jewish Quarterly Review* 18 (1905): 145.

42. *MPME*/S, p. 258; Huling E. Ussery, *Chaucer's Physician: Medicine and Literature in Fourteenth-Century England*, Tulane Studies in English 19 (New Orleans: Department of English, Tulane University, 1971), 55; Weiner, "Note," p. 144.

43. On the development of legal concepts of "Englishness," see Alice Beardwood, "Mercantile Antecedents of the English Naturalization Laws," *Medievalia et Humanistica* 16 (1964): 64–76.

44. C. T. Allmand, "A Note on Denization in Fifteenth Century England," *Medievalia et Humanistica* 17 (1966): 127–28.

45. Edward I financed his household on loans from Italian merchants secured by revenue from wool customs, and Edward III realized that export taxes on wool were the only source of revenue sufficient to finance his claim to French territories; Robert L. Baker, "The English Customs Service, 1307–1343: A Study of Medieval Administration," *Transactions of the American Philosophical Society*, n.s., 51, pt. 6 (Philadelphia, 1961), pp. 11, 34.

46. Beardwood, "Naturalization," p. 72.

47. Frank Barlow notes that among the forty-five medical practitioners listed in *MPME* as living under the Norman kings, one was English, perhaps three were Italian, and the rest were French; *The English Church, 1066–1154* (New York: Longman, 1979), p. 262.

48. On the presence of aliens, especially alien merchants, in England before the conquest, see T. H. Lloyd, *Alien Merchants in England in the High Middle Ages* (New York: St. Martin's Press, 1982), pp. 1–3.

49. *MPME*, pp. 19–21.

50. *MPME*, pp. 63–65; *MPME*/S, p. 260.

51. "Ad regendum Luxouiensem praesulatum Gislebertus cognomento Maminotus regis archiater et capellanus electus est" (*The Ecclesiastical History of Orderic Vitalis*, vol. 3, *Books V and VI*, ed. and trans. Marjorie Chibnall [Oxford: Clarendon Press, 1972], p. 18).

52. Talbot and Hammond note records of Gilbert's English landholdings in the *Doomsday Book*, at least one of which named him as a tenant not of William but of Matilda; *MPME*, p. 64.

53. *The Ecclesiastical History of Orderic Vitalis*, vol. 2, *Books III and IV*, ed. and trans. Marjorie Chibnall (Oxford: Clarendon Press, 1969), pp. 284–93.

54. "Consulti medici inspectione urinae certam mortem praedixere. Quo audito querimonia domum replevit, quod eum praeoccuparet mors emendationem vitae jamdudum meditantem. Resumpto animo, quae Christiani sunt executus est in con-

fessione et viatico" *(Willelmi Malmesbiriensis monachi de gestis regum anglorum libri quin- que,* ed. William Stubbs, Rolls Series 90, vol. 1 [London: HMSO, 1889], p. 337).

55. "Artis medicinae peritissimus erat, sed semetipsum in pontificatu nunquam satis curare poterat. Scientia litterarum et facundia pollebat, diuitiis et deliciis indesi- nenter affluebat, propriae uoluptati et carnis curae nimis seruiebat. Ocio et quieti affatim studebat, ludisque alearum et tesserarum plerunque indulgebat. In cultu aecclesiastico erat piger et negligens, sed ad uenatum auiumque capturam promptus et nimis feruens" *(Orderic,* 3: 20). Chibnall notes the allusion to Luke 4:23: "Physician heal thyself."

56. *MPME,* p. 64.

57. For a context to this monastic disapproval of the vanities of the itinerant Nor- man court, which were said to encourage extravagant male hairdos and flagrant sod- omy, see C. Warren Hollister, "Courtly Culture and Courtly Style in the Anglo-Norman World," *Albion* 20 (1988): 1–17.

58. *MPME,* p. 193; *MPME/S,* p. 268.

59. "Johannes, natione Turonicus, professione medicus. . . . Erat medicus probatis- simus, non scientia sed usu, ut fama, nescio an vera, dispersit. Litteratorum contu- bernio gaudens, ut eorum societate aliquid sibi laudis ascisceret" *(Willelmi Malmesbi- riensis monachi de gestis pontificum anglorum,* ed. N. E. S. A. Hamilton, Rolls Series 52 [1870; reprint, Nendeln: Kraus, 1965], pp. 194–95).

60. On the consternation this move caused, see Barlow, *The English Church, 1066– 1154,* pp. 66–67.

61. *MPME,* p. 193.

62. Ibid., p. 206.

63. Ibid., p. 208. "Deinde rex commisit se manibus cujusdam medici Marchadei, qui, cum conaretur ferrum extrahere, solum lignum extraxit, et sagitta remansit in carne; et cum carnifex ille circumquaque brachium regis minus caute incideret, tan- dem sagittam extraxit" *(Chronica Magistri Rogeri de Houedene,* ed. William Stubbs, Rolls Series 51, vol. 4 [1871; reprint, Nendeln: Kraus, 1964], p. 83 [April 1199]).

64. *MPME,* p. 207.

65. Ibid., pp. 248–49.

66. Ibid., pp. 393–94.

67. *MPME,* pp. 244–45. The same letter recommends Reginald of Stokes, *medicus,* "in artibus et in medicina provecto et experto, quem et conversatio socialis, et circum- specta discretio" *(MPME,* pp. 269–70; *Monumenta Franciscana,* ed. J. S. Brewer, Rolls Series 1, pt. 4 [1858; reprint, Nendeln: Kraus, 1965], p. 113). Also coming from the Continent to serve as Eleanor's physicians were Raymond de Bariamondo *(MPME,* p. 267) and William le Provencal *(MPME,* p. 411).

68. *MPME,* pp. 223–25; *MPME/S,* p. 270.

69. *MPME,* pp. 411–12; *MPME/S,* p. 282.

70. *MPME,* pp. 204–5; *MPME/S,* p. 269.

71. *MPME,* p. 34; *MPME/S,* p. 257.

72. *MPME,* p. 184.

73. Ibid., p. 253.

74. *MPME,* pp. 116–17; *MPME/S,* p. 263.

75. *MPME,* p. 320; *MPME/S,* p. 277.

76. *MPME*, pp. 254–55; *MPME*/S, p. 272. Simon and Philip both married Englishwomen, and Philip had a son, also named Philip. The grandson became involved in a lawsuit in 1321 over whether aliens could inherit exemption from taxes, in this case, exemption granted by Edward to his surgeon, Simon; *Year Books of Edward II: The Eyre of London 14 Edward II, A.D. 1321*, vol. 1, ed. Helen M. Cam, Selden Society 85 (London: B. Quaritch, 1968), pp. lxxiv, lxxxiv, cxxix–cxxx; *Year Books of Edward II: The Eyre of London 14 Edward II, A.D. 1321*, vol. 2, ed. Helen M. Cam, Selden Society 86 (London: B. Quaritch, 1969), pp. 213–17; on the grandson, Williams, *London*, pp. 332–33.

77. *MPME*, pp. 210–11.

78. Ibid., p. 328.

79. *MPME*, p. 215; *MPME*/S, p. 270.

80. Alice Beardwood, *Alien Merchants in England 1350 to 1377: Their Legal Status and Economic Position* (Cambridge, Mass.: Mediaeval Academy of America, 1931), p. 4; Michael Prestwich, "Italian Merchants in Late Thirteenth and Early Fourteenth Century England," in *The Dawn of Modern Banking* (New Haven, Conn.: Yale University Press, 1979), pp. 77–104.

81. *MPME*, pp. 234; *MPME*/S, p. 271; Roger Ellis, "The English Lands and Revenues of Master Pancio da Controne," *Rivista di storia delle scienze mediche e naturali* 43 (1952): 266–74.

82. *MPME*, pp. 48–49.

83. Ibid., p. 204.

84. *MPME*, p. 249; Barbara Harvey, *Living and Dying in England, 1100–1540: The Monastic Experience* (Oxford: Clarendon Press, 1993), p. 233.

85. *MPME*, p. 18.

86. Ibid., p. 248.

87. Ibid., p. 238.

88. Ibid., pp. 249–51.

89. Ibid., p. 98.

90. *MPME*, p. 182; Beardwood, "Naturalization," p. 72.

91. Sylvia L. Thrupp, "Aliens in and around London in the Fifteenth Century," in *Studies in London History Presented to Philip Edmund Jones*, ed. A. E. J. Hollaender and William Kellaway (London: Hodder and Stoughton, 1969), p. 259.

92. *MPME*, p. 18.

93. Ibid., p. 55.

94. Ibid., pp. 96–98.

95. Thrupp, "London," p. 267.

96. *MPME*, p. 252.

97. Ibid., pp. 246–47.

98. *MPME*, pp. 201–2; *MPME*/S, p. 269.

99. *MPME*, p. 240; *Calendar of the Patent Rolls Preserved in the Public Record Office: Edward III*, vol. 16, A.D. 1374–1377 (London: HMSO, 1916), p. 352. Another entry for the same year shows an identical amount granted to Englishman John Bray, also called master, the king's physician; *MPME*, p. 125; *Calendar of the Patent Rolls: Edward III*, p. 354. In 1378 "Master Paul Gabrielis de Ispannia," the king's *fisicus*, last had his pension confirmed by the new king; *Calendar of the Patent Rolls Preserved in the Public Record Office; Richard II*, vol. 1, A.D. 1377–1381 (London: HMSO, 1895), p. 137. Two

days later, Master John Bray was granted £12 annually; *Calendar of the Patent Rolls: Richard II*, 1: 136. By comparison, in the same year John Gosebourn, one of the auditors of the exchequer, was granted £10 a year for life (*Calendar of the Patent Rolls: Richard II*, 1: 136); and John de Masyngham, the king's carpenter, received 10 marks a year (*Calendar of the Patent Rolls: Richard II*, 1: 137). All annuities were received from the exchequer.

100. *MPME*, p. 141; license for John Despanha *medico* to remain in England four years to practice his art; *Calendar of the Patent Rolls Preserved in the Public Record Office; Richard II*, vol. 5, A.D. *1391–1396* (London: HMSO, 1905), p. 36. I was unable to find the reference to "John de Spayne (Despanha)," *MPME*, p. 141, whom Talbot and Hammond conjecture practiced in Essex about 1423 and may have been the same man as John Despanha, who received the license.

101. *MPME*, pp. 34–35.

102. *MPME*, p. 344; Beardwood, "Naturalization," p. 72; Thrupp, "London," p. 261.

103. *MPME/S*, p. 269.

104. The importance of warfare to the development of medical practice should not be exaggerated. Roger Cooter cautioned thus, remarking that "[v]irtually everything that has been written on the subject of war and medicine stresses that the former, for all its horrors, has brought benefit to the latter" ("The Medical Audit of War," in *Companion Encyclopedia of the History of Medicine*, vol. 2, ed. W. F. Bynum and Roy Porter [London: Routledge, 1993], pp. 1541–56, citation on p. 1541). For medieval England, Robert S. Gottfried, in *Doctors and Medicine in Medieval England, 1340–1530* (Princeton, N.J.: Princeton University Press, 1986), has attributed what he sees as the "rise of surgery" in the late Middle Ages to the way in which physicians were "discredited" by their inability to "cure plague," while battlefield "dissections" elevated surgeons. These conclusions are unsupported by any reliable data and ignore the complexities involved in any kind of historical change. On the unsoundness of Gottfried's data, see reviews by Martha Carlin, *Medical History* 31 (1987): 360–62; Faye Getz, *Bulletin of the History of Medicine* 61 (1987): 455–61; and Peter Murray Jones, *Annals of Science* 44 (1987): 542–44. For a thoughtful examination of the complex causes of medical change in medieval society, see McVaugh, *Medicine before the Plague*, esp. p. 245.

105. On English scholars in general, see William J. Courtenay, "English Ties with Continental Learning," in *Schools and Scholars in Fourteenth-Century England* (Princeton, N.J.: Princeton University Press, 1987), pp. 147–67.

106. *MPME*, pp. 372–73; Matthew became prior of the abbey when his brother was named abbot; *MPME*, p. 214; *Gesta Abbatum Monasterii Sancti Albani, a Thoma Walsingham*, ed. Henry Thomas Riley, vol. 1, A.D. *793–1290*. Rolls Series 28, vol. 1, pt. 4 (London: Longman, 1867), p. 194.

107. *MPME*, p. 130.

108. *MPME* p. 91; *MPME/S*, p. 262 ("Hugo of England").

109. *MPME/S*, p. 269.

110. *MPME*, p. 113; *MPME/S*, p. 263.

111. *MPME*, p. 133; A. B. Emden, *A Biographical Register of the University of Cambridge to 1500* (Cambridge: Cambridge University Press, 1963), p. 139; hereafter *BRUC*.

112. *MPME*, p. 147. In general, Rosamond J. Mitchell, *John Free: From Bristol to Rome in the Fifteenth Century* (London: Longman, 1955).

113. *MPME*, p. 398; *MPME/S*, p. 281; *BRUC*, pp. 292–93.

114. On learning at the *studium curiae* under papal patronage, see Agostino Paravicini Bagliani, *Medicina e scienze della natura alla corte dei papi del duecento* (Spoleto: Centro Italiano di Studi Sull'alto Medioevo, 1991).

115. Paravicini Bagliani, *Medicina e scienze della natura*, pp. 261–64, 403–4; *MPME*, pp. 190–91; Danielle Jacquart, *Dictionnaire biographique des médecins en France au moyen âge: Supplément* (Geneva: Librairie Droz, 1979), pp. 186–87.

116. *MPME*, pp. 92–93; *MPME*/S, p. 263; Paravicini Bagliani, *Medicina e scienze della natura*, pp. 261–64, 399–405.

117. *MPME*, p. 273; *Calendar of the Liberate Rolls Preserved in the Public Record Office, Henry III*, vol. 3, A.D. *1245–1251* (London: HMSO, 1937), p. 60.

118. *MPME*, p. 70. Arnald of Villanova was born in 1240 and died in 1311; *Dictionary of Scientific Biography*, s.v. "Arnald of Villanova."

119. *MPME*, p. 87; *MPME*/S, p. 261; an edition of the text in Latin and Middle English, along with important introductory material, is *A Latin Technical Phlebotomy and Its Middle English Translation*, ed. Linda E. Voigts and Michael R. McVaugh, *Transactions of the American Philosophical Society* 74, pt. 2 (Philadelphia, 1984).

120. G. E. Trease, "The Spicers and Apothecaries of the Royal Household in the Reigns of Henry III, Edward I and Edward II," *Nottingham Mediaeval Studies* 3 (1959): 24.

121. *MPME*, p. 237. The malady afflicted other members of the household. Gilbert Talbot was ill in March with Pancio, and with John Lestraunge, described as the late king's yeoman. Payment was ordered from the exchequer to John's attendants and "the physicians who came to him" (*Calendar of Close Rolls Preserved in the Public Record Office: Edward III, A.D. 1327–1330* [London: HMSO, 1896], pp. 432–33).

122. *MPME*, p. 92; *MPME*, p. 130.

123. *MPME*, p. 159; *MPME*/S, p. 266; *BRUC*, p. 341: John Kun; and *BRUC*, p. 342: John Kyme. See also Scotsman John de Lyle, who studied medicine at Paris in the middle of the fifteenth century; *MPME*, p. 164; *MPME*/S, p. 266.

124. *MPME*, p. 327; *MPME*/S, p. 277.

125. *MPME*, p. 336; *MPME*/S, p. 278.

126. In obsidione castrorum necessarii sunt medici et maxime vulnera curare scientes. The letter was addressed to Ralph, bishop of Chichester, and was written some time before 1230; *MPME*/S, p. 277.

127. Kealey, *Medicus*, p. 95.

128. *MPME*, p. 206.

129. Ibid., p. 330.

130. *MPME*, p. 126; *Dictionary of National Biography*, s.v. William de Valence.

131. *MPME*, p. 111.

132. S. J. Lang, "John Bradmore and His Book *Philomena,*" *Social History of Medicine* 5 (1992): 122.

133. *MPME*, pp. 359–60, *MPME*/S, p. 279.

134. *MPME*, p. 210.

135. *MPME*, p. 351; *MPME*/S, pp. 278–79; George Gask, "The Medical Services of Henry the Fifth's Campaign of the Somme in 1415," *in Essays in the History of Medicine* (London: Butterworth, 1950), pp. 94–102.

136. Faye Marie Getz, "The Faculty of Medicine before 1500," in *The History of the University of Oxford*, vol. 2, *Late Medieval Oxford*, ed. Jeremy Catto and Ralph Evans (Oxford: Clarendon Press, 1992), pp. 393–94.

137. *MPME*, p. 351; Sylvia L. Thrupp, *The Merchant Class of Medieval London 1300– 1500* (Chicago: University of Chicago Press, 1948), pp. 260, 383.

138. Wickersheimer, *Dictionnaire biographique*, p. 612; *MPME/S*, p. 271.

139. *MPME*, p. 381; *MPME/S*, p. 281; *Dictionary of Scientific Biography*, s.v. "William the Englishman.

140. *MPME/S*, p. 283.

Chapter III
The Medieval English Medical Text

1. See especially Linda E. Voigts, "Medical Prose," in *Middle English Prose: A Critical Guide to Major Authors and Genres*, ed. A. S. G. Edwards (New Brunswick, N.J.: Rutgers University Press, 1984), pp. 315–35; Voigts, "Scientific and Medical Books," in *Book Production and Publishing in Britain, 1375–1475*, ed. Jeremy Griffiths and Derek Pearsall (Cambridge: Cambridge University Press, 1989), pp. 345–402; Rossell Hope Robbins, "Medical Manuscripts in Middle English," *Speculum* 45 (1970): 393–415. The most important resource for the field is a database of information on Old and Middle English scientific and medical texts prepared by Linda Ehrsam Voigts and Patricia Deery Kurtz. It will appear on CD-ROM and in book form. Preliminary findings of the database are presented in Voigts, "Multitudes of Middle English Medical Manuscripts, or the Englishing of Science and Medicine," in *Manuscript Sources of Medieval Medicine: A Book of Essays*, ed. Margaret R. Schleissner (New York: Garland Publishing, 1995), pp. 183–95.

2. *Popular Medicine in Thirteenth-Century England: Introduction and Texts*, ed. Tony Hunt (Cambridge, England: D. S. Brewer, 1990), which is an erudite study of pharmaceutical literature; in general, William Rothwell, "The Role of French in Thirteenth-Century England," *Bulletin of the John Rylands University Library* 58 (1975–76): 445–66.

3. For example, London, British Library, Sloane MS 6, from the early fifteenth century, contains a partial English translation of Galen's *De ingenio sanitatis* and translations of the *Isagoge* of Johannitius and sections of the *Liber regius* of Haly Abbas, all university Latin medical texts; Faye Marie Getz, "The *Method of Healing* in Middle English," in *Galen's Method of Healing: Proceedings of the 1982 Galen Symposium*, ed. Fridolf Kudlien and Richard J. Durling (Leiden: E. J. Brill, 1991), pp. 147–56.

4. Faye Marie Getz, ed., *Healing and Society in Medieval England: A Middle English Translation of the Pharmaceutical Writings of Gilbertus Anglicus* (Madison: University of Wisconsin Press, 1991), pp. xli–xlviii, lxviii-lxxii; in general, Malcolm B. Parkes, "The Influence of the Concepts of *Ordinatio* and *Compilatio* on the Development of the Book," in *Medieval Learning and Literature: Essays Presented to Richard William Hunt*, ed. J. J. G. Alexander and M. T. Gibson (Oxford: Clarendon Press, 1976), pp. 115–41.

5. *Hippocratic Writings*, ed. G. E. R. Lloyd (New York: Penguin Books, 1978), p. 9.

6. G. E. R. Lloyd, "The Criticism of Magic and the Inquiry Concerning Nature," in *Magic, Reason and Experience: Studies in the Origin and Development of Greek Science* (Cambridge: Cambridge University Press, 1979), pp. 10–58; Ludwig Edelstein, "Greek Medicine in Its Relation to Religion and Magic," in *Ancient Medicine: Selected Papers of*

Ludwig Edelstein, ed. Owsei Temkin and C. Lilian Temkin (Baltimore, Md.: The Johns Hopkins University Press, 1967), pp. 205–46.

7. Edelstein, "The Hippocratic Physician," in *Ancient Medicine*, pp. 87–110.

8. "Tradition in Medicine," in *Hippocratic Writings*, pp. 70–86. On medieval understanding of Hippocratic ideas of medical progress, see Chiara Crisciani, "History, Novelty, and Progress in Scholastic Medicine," *Osiris*, 2d ser., 6 (1990): 118–39.

9. Gordon L. Miller, "Literacy and the Hippocratic Art: Reading, Writing, and Epistemology in Ancient Greek Medicine," *Journal of the History of Medicine* 45 (1990): 11–40; Iain M. Lonie, "Literacy and the Development of Hippocratic Medicine," in *Formes de pensée dans la Collection Hippocratique*, ed. F. Lasserre and P. Mudry (Geneva: Librairie Droz, 1983), pp. 145–61.

10. These arguments are especially forceful in the treatise "The Sacred Disease," in *Hippocratic Writings*, pp. 237–51.

11. Gerhard Baader, "Die Tradition des Corpus Hippocraticum im europäischen Mittelalter," *Sudhoffs Archiv* Beiheft 27 (1989): 409–19; Pearl Kibre, *Hippocrates Latinus: Repertorium of Hippocratic Writings in the Latin Middle Ages*, rev. ed. (New York: Fordham University Press, 1985). For late-medieval knowledge about Hippocrates, "a parfite man in vertues and vsed experience & reason togedir," see *The Dicts and Sayings of the Philosophers*, ed. Curt F. Bühler, Early English Text Society, o.s., 211 (1941; reprint, London: Oxford University Press, 1961), pp. 44–51 (citation on p. 45).

12. Owsei Temkin, "Galen's Ideal Philosopher," in *Hippocrates in a World of Pagans and Christians* (Baltimore, Md.: The Johns Hopkins University Press, 1991), pp. 47–50.

13. Jonathan Barnes, "Galen on Logic and Therapy," in *Galen's Method of Healing: Proceedings of the 1982 Galen Symposium*, ed. Fridolf Kudlein and Richard J. Durling (Leiden: E. J. Brill, 1991), pp. 50–102 esp. p. 51, n. 7.

14. Owsei Temkin, "The Portrait of an Ideal," in *Galenism: Rise and Decline of a Medical Philosophy* (Ithaca: Cornell University Press, 1973), pp. 10–50.

15. The ability to read at least a little Greek never disappeared from the West entirely; see Mary Catherine Bodden, "Evidence for Knowledge of Greek in Anglo-Saxon England," *Anglo-Saxon England* 17 (1988): 217–46; Montague Rhodes James, "Greek Manuscripts in England before the Renaissance," *The Library*, n.s., 7 (1927): 337–53. For late-medieval knowledge of Galen, who "lerned phesyk of a womman that was called Cleupare [Cleopatra], which taught him and shewed many goode herbes, namely for sekenesse of wommen," see *Dicts and Sayings*, pp. 256–61.

16. See esp. *Dictionary of Scientific Biography*, s.v. "Hunayn ibn Ishaq"; Manfred Ullmann, *Islamic Medicine* (Edinburgh: Edinburgh University Press, 1978); Fuat Sezgin, "Hunain b. Ishaq," in *Geschichte des arabischen Schrifttums* (Leiden: E. J. Brill, 1970), 3; 247–56.

17. Nancy G. Siraisi, *Avicenna in Renaissance Italy* (Princeton, N.J.: Princeton University Press, 1987); G. Anawati, "Medicine," in *The Cambridge History of Islam*, ed. P. M. Holt, Ann K. S. Lambton, and Bernard Lewis (Cambridge: Cambridge University Press, 1970), 2;765–79 ; F. Gabrieli, "The Transmission of Learning," in *The Cambridge History of Islam*, 2:851–68; Ullmann, *Islamic Medicine*, pp. 152–6.

18. Charles S. F. Burnett, "Some Comments on the Translating of Works from Arabic into Latin in the Mid-Twelfth Century," in *Orientalische Kultur und Europäisches Mittelalter*, ed. Albert Zimmermann, Miscellanea Mediaevalia 17 (Berlin: Walter de

Gruyter, 1985), pp. 161–71; Marie-Thérèse D'Alverny, "Translations and Translators," in *Renaissance and Renewal in the Twelfth Century*, ed. Robert L. Benson and Giles Constable, with Carol D. Lanham (Cambridge, Mass.: Harvard University Press, 1982), pp. 421–62.

19. Paul Oskar Kristeller, "The School of Salerno: Its Development and Contribution to the History of Learning," *Bulletin of the History of Medicine* 17 (1945): 138–94; Herbert Bloch, *Monte Cassino in the Middle Ages*, vol. 1 (Cambridge, Mass.: Harvard University Press, 1986), pp. 98–110; *Dictionary of Scientific Biography*, s.v. "Constantine the African."

20. For a summary with bibliography of Western medicine before and shortly after the introduction of Latin translations of Arabic sources, see Danielle Jacquart, "The Introduction of Arabic Medicine into the West: The Question of Etiology," in *Health, Disease and Healing in Medieval Culture*, ed. Sheila Campbell, Bert Hall, and David Klausner (New York: St. Martin's Press, 1992), pp. 186–95.

21. Mary F. Wack, *Lovesickness in the Middle Ages: The* Viaticum *and Its Commentaries* (Philadelphia: University of Pennsylvania Press, 1990), esp. pp. 34–38.

22. Dorothee Metlitzki, *The Matter of Araby in Medieval England* (New Haven, Conn.: Yale University Press, 1977), pp. 3–12.

23. J. A. Weisheipl, "Science in the Thirteenth Century," in *The History of the University of Oxford*, vol. 1, *The Early Oxford Schools*, ed. J. I. Catto and T. A. R. Evans (Oxford: Clarendon Press, 1984), pp. 435 ff.

24. Metlitzki, *The Matter of Araby*, pp. 13–55; and the essays in *Adelard of Bath: An English Scientist and Arabist of the Early Twelfth Century*, ed. Charles Burnett (London: The Warburg Institute, 1987).

25. On whether medicine was properly a graduate or an undergraduate subject, see Faye Marie Getz, "The Faculty of Medicine before 1500," in *The History of the University of Oxford*, vol. 2, *Late Medieval Oxford*, ed. Jeremy Catto and Ralph Evans (Oxford: Clarendon Press, 1992), pp. 388–89.

26. *Alfred of Sareshel's Commentary on the* Metheora *of Aristotle*, ed. James K. Otte (Leiden: E. J. Brill, 1988), p. 4.

27. *Alfred of Sareshel (Alfredus Anglicus), De motu cordis*, ed. Clemens Baeumker, *Beiträge zur Geschichte der Philosophie des Mittelalters* 23 (1923); pts. 1–2.

28. A modern medical evaluation of Gilbert's writings, along with summaries of various passages from the *Compendium*, is Henry E. Handerson, *Gilbertus Anglicus: Medicine of the Thirteenth Century* (Cleveland, Ohio: Cleveland Medical Library Association, 1918).

29. *MPME*, pp. 58–60; *MPME/S*, p. 259.

30. Agostino Paravicini Bagliani, *Medicina e scienze della natura alla corte dei papi nel duecento* (Spoleto: Centro Italiano di Studi Sull'Alto Medioevo, 1991).

31. *MPME*, p. 59.

32. Gilbertus Anglicus, *Compendium medicine* (Lyons: J. Saccon for V. de Portonariis, 1510), fol. 47. Gilbert's citation is to Richard's work on urines, which he does not name, but which is probably the so-called *Regula de urinis*, usually appearing among the collection attributed to Richard called *Micrologus*; *MPME*, pp. 270–71. Numerous manuscripts survive and are cited in Lynn Thorndike and Pearl Kibre, *A Catalogue of Incipits of Mediaeval Scientific Writings in Latin* (London: Mediaeval Academy of America, 1963), cols. 223, 1247, hereafter TK; and *MPME*, p. 271 n. 3. The most

complete discussion of Richard's manuscript tradition is in Ernest Wickersheimer, *Dictionnaire biographique des médecins en France au moyen âge* (Paris: Librairie E. Droz, 1936), pp. 694–98; and Danielle Jacquart, *Dictionnaire biographique des médecins en France au moyen âge: Supplément* (Geneva: Librairie Droz, 1979), pp. 256–57.

33. Paravicini Bagliani, *Medicina e scienze della natura*, pp. 17–20, who examines assertions made in *MPME*, pp. 58–60.

34. *The Canterbury Tales, General Prologue*, in *The Works of Geoffrey Chaucer*, ed. F. N. Robinson, 2d ed. (Boston: Houghton Mifflin, 1957), p. 21 (1. 434).

35. Vermes aliquando creantur in auribus precipue saniosis et vlcerosis . . . aliquando autem vermis sive aliud reptile in aurem intrat (Gilbertus, *Compendium*, fol. 147).

36. Tinnitus aurium fit ex ventositate inclusa in cavernis aurium non habente exitum propter grossitudinem suam (ibid., fol. 147v).

37. On Gilbert's pharmaceutical system, see Getz, *Healing and Society*, pp. xxxvii–xli.

38. Gilbertus, *Compendium*, fol. 178.

39. Ibid., fol. 178v.

40. Ibid., fol. 16v.

41. In the popular Middle English translation: "I haue taken litel of emperykes and of charmes, of the whiche thinges plente is founden in Gilbertyn and in Thesauro Pauperum [of Petrus Hispanus]" (*The Cyrurgie of Guy de Chauliac*, ed. Margaret Ogden, Early English Text Society 265, [London and New York: Oxford University Press, 1971], pp. 533–34); in the original Latin: "Empericas et incantaciones parum acceptavi, de quibus in Gilbertina et Thesauro pauperum copia invenitur multa" (*Guigonis de Caulhiaco (Guy de Chauliac): Inventarium sive Chirurgia Magna*, vol. 1, ed. Michael R. McVaugh [Leiden: E. J. Brill, 1997], p. 391).

42. On charms to heal wounds, and on their acceptability to the clergy, see Lea T. Olsan, "Latin Charms of Medieval England: Verbal Healing in a Christian Oral Tradition," *Oral Tradition* 7 (1992): 116–42.

43. Gilbertus, *Compendium*, fol. 88. Recounted in part by Handerson, *Gilbertus*, p. 27. The charm must have been popular in Guy de Chauliac's time as well. He described the various medical and surgical sects of his day. The second worst (before "women and idiots") was the crusading orders, "alle knyghtes of Saxoun and of men folowynge batailles, the whiche procuren or helen alle woundes with coniurisouns and drynkes and with oyle and wolle and a cole leef, foundynge ham therfore vppon that, that God putte his vertu in herbes, wordes and stones" (*Cyrurgie of Guy*, p. 10; *Guigonis*, p. 7). For similar charms for wounds see Lea T. Olsan, "Latin Charms in British Library, MS Royal 12.B.XXV," *Manuscripta* 33 (1989): 119–28.

44. Gilbertus, *Compendium*, fol. 142; Leviticus 14:49–53.

45. Gilbertus, *Compendium*, fol. 16v.

46. Ibid., fol. 20v.

47. London, Wellcome Institute Library, MS 547: "medicus est artifex sensibilis . . ." (fol. 105, col. 2). The entire commentary covers fols. 104–45v.

48. C. H. Talbot, *Medicine in Medieval England* (London: Oldbourne, 1967), p. 73.

49. Found in book 4, chap. 7, in modern English translation in *The Surgery of Theodoric*, trans. Eldridge Campbell and James Colton, vol. 2 (New York: Appleton-Century-Crofts, 1960), p. 211.

50. Identified and edited in Middle English in Getz, *Healing and Society*; it was one of the most widely copied Middle English medical texts. See Voigts, "Multitudes," p. 189.

51. Getz, *Healing and Society*, p. lv; Oxford M.D. Simon Bredon once owned a copy of the *Compendium*, now Oxford, Merton College MS N. 3. 9 (Coxe MS 226).

52. For the construction of medical compendia, see Luke C. Demaitre, "Scholasticism in Compendia of Practical Medicine, 1250–1450," *Manuscripta* 20 (1976): 81–95.

53. John Gaddesden, *Rosa anglica practica a capite ad pedes* (Pavia, 1492), fol. 1: "erit pro pauperibus divitibus cirurgicis et medicis."

54. Ibid., fol. 1.

55. Ibid., fol. 77v.

56. Ibid., fol. 85.

57. Ibid., fol. 94.

58. Ibid., fols. 116v–17.

59. Ibid., fol. 171.

60. H. P. Cholmeley, *John of Gaddesden and the Rosa Medicinae* (Oxford: Clarendon Press, 1912), pp. 147–84.

61. Gaddesden, *Rosa*, fol. 50. See also Peter Murray Jones, "John of Arderne and the Mediterranean Tradition of Scholastic Surgery," in *Practical Medicine from Salerno to the Black Death*, ed. Luis García-Ballester, Roger French, Jon Arrizabalaga, and Andrew Cunningham (Cambridge: Cambridge University Press, 1994), p. 308, which describes a similar tendency to vernacular glossing by a surgeon.

62. Peter Murray Jones has written several excellent studies of Arderne and his writings; see esp. "Mediterranean," pp. 289–321.

63. Arderne wrote that he treated Henry Blakburn, treasurer of the Black Prince's household; Jones, "Mediterranean," p. 296 n 17. Gaddesden was in Edward's service; *MPME*, pp. 149–50.

64. On translations of Arderne see Peter Murray Jones, "Four Middle English Translations of John of Arderne," in *Latin and Vernacular: Studies in Late Medieval Manuscripts*, ed. Alastair Minnis (Wolfeboro, N.H.: D. S. Brewer, 1989), pp. 61–89. On the illustrations, see Jones, " 'Sicut hic depingitur . . .': John of Arderne and English Medical Illustration in the 14th and 15th Centuries," in *Die Kunst und das Studium der Natur vom 14. zum 16. Jahrhundert*, ed. Wolfram Prinz and Andreas Beyer (Weinheim: VCH, 1987), pp. 103–26, 379–92.

65. On the patients' identities, see Jones, "Mediterranean," pp. 295–96.

66. Bredon's *Trifolium* is in Oxford, Bodleian Library, Digby MS 160, fols. 102–222v; TK 761. Its contents are examined and brushed off by C. H. Talbot, in "Simon Bredon (c. 1300–1372), Physician, Mathematician and Astronomer," *British Journal for the History of Science* 1 (1962–63): 19–30, who found the work "excruciatingly dull" (p. 22). The identification of the text as Bredon's and the date 1380 appear on fol. 102, possibly in Digby's hand. For Bredon's life, see *MPME*, pp. 320–22, and *MPME*/S, p. 277. On Bredon's arithmetic, see J. D. North, "Astronomy and Mathematics," in *The History of the University of Oxford*, vol. 2, *Late Medieval Oxford*, ed. Jeremy Cato and Ralph Evans (Oxford: Clarendon Press, 1992), "Faculty of Medicine," pp. 136–37; and Getz, pp. 392–93.

67. Incipit: *Urina secundum Constantinum et Theophilum est colamentum sanguinis.*

68. Other texts in the same manuscript are an excerpt from Guy de Chauliac's surgery, fol. 22: *Quoniam secundum Galeinum medicorum* (TK 1301); and the *Speculum* of Arnald of Villanova, fol. 46: *Speculum arnoldi super johannicium. medicina est scientia cognoscendi* (TK 857).

69. Outlined by Michael R. McVaugh, "Quantified Medical Theory and Practice at Fourteenth-Century Montpellier," *Bulletin of the History of Medicine* 43 (1969): 397–413; also Edith Sylla, "Medieval Quantifications of Qualities: The 'Merton School,' " *Archive for History of Exact Sciences* 8 (1971): 20–24; McVaugh, "An Early Discussion of Medicinal Degrees at Montpellier by Henry of Winchester," *Bulletin of the History of Medicine* 49 (1975): 57–71; *Arnaldi de Villanova, Opera Medica Omnia II: Aphorismi de Gradibus*, ed. Michael R. McVaugh (Granada-Barcelona: Seminarium Historiae Medicae Granatensis, 1975).

70. "Intencio mea in hoc opusculo fuit iuxta triplex regimen" (Digby 160, fol. 102; TK 761).

71. Pliny, *Natural History, with an English Translation in Ten Volumes*, vol. 8, ed. W. H. S. Jones, Loeb Classical Library (Cambridge, Mass.: Harvard University Press, 1975), pp. 200–201; Faye Marie Getz, "To Prolong Life and Promote Health: Baconian Alchemy and Pharmacy in the English Learned Tradition," in *Health, Disease and Healing in Medieval Culture*, ed. Sheila Campbell, Bert Hall, and David Klausner (New York: St. Martin's Press, 1992), p. 143.

72. Pliny's ideas about the supernatural are not our own. He cautioned against the use of "portentous magic" [magica portenta] in remedies but assigned to peony the property of preventing "the mocking delusions that the Fauns bring on us in our sleep"; Pliny, *Natural History, with an English Translation in Ten Volumes*, vol. 7, ed. W. H. S. Jones, Loeb Classical Library (Cambridge, Mass.: Harvard University Press, 1966), pp. 154–57.

73. On Pliny in the ancient world, and on his views of Greek physicians, see Roger French, *Ancient Natural History: Histories of Nature* (London: Routledge, 1994), pp. 223–25. On Pliny's methodology of "text criticising text," see G. E. R. Lloyd, *Science, Folklore and Ideology* (Cambridge: Cambridge University Press, 1983), p. 149. On medieval encyclopedias in general and the survival of Pliny's in particular, see Marjorie Chibnall, "Pliny's *Natural History* and the Middle Ages," in *Empire and Aftermath: Silver Latin II*, ed. T. A. Dorey (London: Routledge and Kegan Paul, 1975), pp. 57–78. On the humanistic aspects of this reverence for Pliny and the Latin language, see Jerome J. Bylebyl, "Medicine, Philosophy, and Humanism in Renaissance Italy," in *Science and the Arts in the Renaissance*, ed. John W. Shirley and F. David Hoeniger (Washington, D.C.: The Folger Shakespeare Library, 1985), pp. 27–49, esp. p. 35.

74. Paul Abelson, *The Seven Liberal Arts: A Study in Mediaeval Culture* (New York: Russell and Russell, 1906, reissued 1965), pp. 1–10. A more thorough study with citations from primary sources is Friedmar Kühnert, *Allgemeinbildung und Fachbildung in der Antike* (Berlin: Akademie-Verlag, 1961); see also M. L. Clarke, *Higher Education in the Ancient World* (London: Routledge and Kegan Paul, 1971), esp. 109–18.

75. On the medicine of Varro and Celsus as "part of the general knowledge that every true paterfamilias was supposed to possess," see H. I. Marrou, *History of Education in Antiquity*, trans. George Lamb (New York: Sheed and Ward, 1956), p. 254. See also *Marcus Porcius Cato on Agriculture, Marcus Terentius Varro on Agriculture*, trans. William

Davis Hooper, rev. Harrison Boyd Ash, Loeb Classical Library (Cambridge, Mass.: Harvard University Press, 1954).

76. Talbot, *Medicine in Medieval England*, pp. 9–23; Nancy G. Siraisi, *Medieval and Early Renaissance Medicine: An Introduction to Knowledge and Practice* (Chicago: University of Chicago Press, 1990), pp. 6–11; M. L. Cameron, "The Sources of Medical Knowledge in Anglo-Saxon England," *Anglo-Saxon England* 11 (1983): 135–55. Cameron called attention to a number of writings that could have been known in monastic libraries by the middle of the eighth century, including Latin epitomes of Dioscorides, Oribasius, and Alexander of Tralles, as well as the Latin writers Marcellus of Bordeaux, Cassius Felix, Caelius Aurelianus, Pliny, and Isidore of Seville (pp. 137–42).

77. *Cassiodori Senatoris Institutiones*, ed. R. A. B. Mynors (Oxford: Clarendon Press, 1937), pp. 78–79 (bk. 1, chap. 31), relevant parts translated in Talbot, *Medicine in Medieval England*, pp. 13–14; also Anne F. Dawtry, "The *Modus Medendi* and the Benedictine Order in Anglo-Norman England," *Studies in Church History* 19 (1982): 25–38.

78. On the medieval tradition of paterfamiliar literature, see Volker Zimmermann, *Rezeption und Rolle der Heilkunde in landessprachigen handschriftlichen Kompendien des Spätmittelalters* (Stuttgart: Franz Steiner Verlag Wiesbaden, 1986), esp. "Die Rezeption der Heilkunde aus den Kompendien in die 'Hausväterliteratur'," pp. 120–26.

79. Pliny noted that charms and prayers were believed to be effective by many great men, including Cato, and persuaded himself that their power was in the end a matter of personal opinion; Pliny, *Natural History* 8: 8–23.

80. "Infirmorm cura ante omnia et super omnia adhibenda est, ut sicut revera Christo ita eis serviatur." Scriptural citations to Matt. 25:36 and Matt. 25:40 follow; *The Rule of St. Benedict: In Latin and English with Notes*, ed. Timothy Fry et al. (Collegeville, Minn.: The Liturgical Press, 1981), pp. 234–35 (chap. 35).

81. *Bedae Venerabilis Opera: Pars VI, Opera Didascalica, 1*, ed. Charles W. Jones, Corpus Christianorum Series Latina, vol. 123A (Turnoholti: Typographi Brepols, 1975), xi, pp. 174, 187. Bede did not treat medicine per se, only plague, which he considered among meteorological phenomena (p. 233; chap. 37).

82. The best general description of the location and nature of medical material in Old English remains Linda E. Voigts, "Anglo-Saxon Plant Remedies and the Anglo-Saxons," *Isis* 70 (1979): 250–68.

83. See, for example, Maria Amalia D'Aronco, "The Botanical Lexicon of the Old English *Herbarium*," *Anglo-Saxon England* 17 (1988): 15–33.

84. For a painstaking study of the variety of sources used by the copyists of Anglo-Saxon remedy books, see M. L. Cameron, "Making a *Leechbook*," in *Anglo-Saxon Medicine* (Cambridge: Cambridge University Press, 1993), pp. 74–99. A study of archaeological and textual evidence for native pagan and Continental elements in women's medicine is Audrey Meaney, "Women, Witchcraft and Magic in Anglo-Saxon England," in *Superstition and Popular Medicine in Anglo-Saxon England*, ed. D. G. Scragg (Manchester: Centre for Anglo-Saxon Studies, 1989), pp. 9–40.

85. Audrey Meaney examines the physical aspects of manuscript assembly, including the use of scraps of parchment, in "Variant Versions of Old English Medical Remedies and the Compilation of Bald's *Leechbook*," *Anglo-Saxon England* 13 (1984): 235–68.

86. Wilfrid Bonser, *The Medical Background of Anglo-Saxon England: A Study in History, Psychology, and Folklore* (London: Wellcome Historical Medical Library, 1963), pp. 13–21.

87. Bonser, *Medical Background*, pp. 24–27; Cameron, *Anglo-Saxon Medicine*, pp. 30–64. Cameron's chapter "Compilations in Latin," pp. 48–58, is a necessary reminder that medical material from Anglo-Saxon England survives not only in Old English but also in Latin.

88. Cameron, *Anglo-Saxon Medicine*, pp. 130–58 (with numerous examples in modern English translation); Bonser, *Medical Background*, pp. 117–263 (more wide-ranging, covering chronicles, laws, accounts of demonic possession, and healing with relics; also with numerous translations); Olsan, "Latin Charms of Medieval England" (explores charms' cultural meaning and complexity).

89. Cameron, *Anglo-Saxon Medicine*, pp. 174–84 (translations into modern English); Bonser, *Medical Background*, pp. 264–70 (translations also).

90. Cameron, *Anglo-Saxon Medicine*, pp. 159–73 (translations; considers bloodletting and its theory); Bonser, *Medical Background*, pp. 98–108 (translations).

91. Voigts, "Anglo-Saxon Plant Remedies"; Cameron, *Anglo-Saxon Medicine*, pp. 100–116; Bonser, *Medical Background*, pp. 306–46. Material on herbal healing is also scattered throughout other parts of the two books.

92. N. R. Ker, *Catalogue of Manuscripts Containing Anglo-Saxon* (Oxford: Clarendon Press, 1957), no. 264 (pp. 332–33).

93. "Bald habet hunc librum Cild quem conscribere iussit." Cited by J. N. Adams and Marilyn Deegan, "Bald's *Leechbook* and the *Physica Plinii*," *Anglo-Saxon England* 21 (1992); 87.

94. Adams and Deegan, "Bald's *Leechbook*," pp. 88–89; Meaney, "Variant Versions," p. 251. The Leechbook of Bald was edited by Deegan for her doctoral dissertation (Manchester, 1988) and will be published by the Early English Text Society (Adams and Deegan, "Bald's *Leechbook*," p. 89, n 19). The text was published in 1865 as vol. 2 of *Leechdoms, Wortcunning and Starcraft of Early England*, ed. Thomas Oswald Cockayne (reprint, London: Holland Press, 1961).

95. Meaney, "Variant Versions," pp. 236–37; Adams and Deegan, "Bald's *Leechbook*," p. 88; Cameron, *Anglo-Saxon Medicine*, pp. 35–42, describes its contents.

96. Meaney, "Variant Versions," p. 236.

97. M. L. Cameron, "Bald's *Leechbook* and Cultural Interactions in Anglo-Saxon England," *Anglo-Saxon England* 19 (1990); 5.

98. The most thorough source study is M. L. Cameron, "Bald's *Leechbook*: Its Sources and Their Use in Its Compilation," *Anglo-Saxon England* 12 (1983): 153–82, with some translations.

99. Olsan, "Latin Charms of Medieval England," pp. 118–19.

100. Adams and Deegan, "Bald's *Leechbook*," pp. 112–13.

101. Audrey Meaney, "King Alfred and His Secretariat," *Parergon* 11 (1975): 16–23; Malcolm B. Parkes, "The Palaeography of the Parker Manuscript of the Chronicle, Laws and Sedulius, and Historiography at Winchester in the Late Ninth and Tenth Centuries," *Anglo-Saxon England* 5 (1976): 149–71; J. D. A. Ogilvy, *Books Known to Anglo-Saxon Writers from Aldhelm to Alcuin (670–804)* (Cambridge, Mass.: Mediaeval Academy of America, 1936); *Codices Latini Antiquiores: A Palaeographical Guide to Latin Manu-*

scripts Prior to the Ninth Century, 2d ed., ed. E. A. Lowe, rev. by Virginia Brown (Oxford: Clarendon Press, 1972).

102. "Isidore of Seville: The Medical Writings: An English Translation with an Introduction and Commentary," ed. William D. Sharpe, *Transactions of the American Philosophical Society,* n.s., vol. 54, pt. 2 (Philadelphia, 1964), p. 64; also John A. Alford, "Medicine in the Middle Ages: The Theory of a Profession," *Centennial Review* 23 (1979): 381.

103. "Hinc est quod Medicina secunda Philosophia dicitur. Vtraque enim disciplina totum hominem sibi vindicat. Nam sicut per illam anima, ita per hanc corpus curatur" (Isidore of Seville, *Etimologías: Edición Bilingüe,* vol. 1, ed. and trans. José Oroz Reta and Manuel-A. Marcos Casquero [Madrid: Biblioteca de Autores Cristianos, 1982], p. 506; *De sensu* 1.436a). See also Siraisi, *Medieval and Early Renaissance Medicine,* pp. 2–4.

104. R. W. Hunt, "The Scientist," in *The Schools and the Cloister: The Life and Writings of Alexander Nequam (1157–1217),* ed. and rev. Margaret Gibson (Oxford: Clarendon Press, 1984), pp. 67–83; manuscripts and printed excerpts pp. 134–36.

105. *On the Properties of Things: John Trevisa's Translation of* Bartholomaeus Anglicus De Proprietatibus Rerum, *A Critical Text,* ed. M. C. Seymour et al., 3 vols. (Oxford: Clarendon Press, 1975–88). These editors use the 1601 printed edition of *De proprietatibus rerum* (Frankfurt am Main: Minerva G. M. B. H., 1964), which I also use for comparison.

106. M. C. Seymour et al., *Bartholomaeus Anglicus and His Encyclopedia* (Aldershot: Variorum, 1992), p. 10. This book provides further endnotes to those supplied in vol. 3 of *On the Properties of Things.*

107. *Bartholomaeus Anglicus and His Encyclopedia,* pp. 23–25; Getz, "Faculty of Medicine," p. 376.

108. *Bartholomaeus Anglicus and His Encyclopedia,* pp. 87–96 (prepared by Malcolm Andrew).

109. *On the Properties of Things,* notes in vol. 3, p. 87 (prepared by Malcolm Andrew).

110. *De proprietatibus rerum,* p. 286; *On the Properties of Things,* 1; 352–53.

111. Mirfield has been the subject of several studies, the first mentioned most useful: *Johannes de Mirfeld of St Bartholomew's, Smithfield: His Life and Works,* ed. Percival Horton-Smith Hartley and Harold Richard Aldridge (Cambridge: Cambridge University Press, 1936); *John of Mirfield (d. 1407), Surgery: A Translation of his* Breviarium Bartholomei, *Part IX,* ed. James B. Colton (New York: Hafner, 1969); Faye Marie Getz, "John Mirfield and the *Breviarium Bartholomei*: The Medical Writings of a Clerk at St Bartholomew's Hospital in the Later Fourteenth Century," *Society for the Social History of Medicine Bulletin* 37 (1985): 24–26. I have adopted the spelling "Mirfield" as opposed to the less usual "Mirfeld," because the former is the common spelling of the Yorkshire town of the family's origin.

112. On the hospital, see Martha Carlin, "Medieval English Hospitals," in *The Hospital in History,* ed. Lindsay Granshaw and Roy Porter (London: Routledge, 1989), p. 33; and Carole Rawcliffe, "The Hospitals of Later Medieval London," *Medical History* 28 (1984): 2.

113. *Johannes de Mirfeld,* pp. 11–12, 16, 17 n. 1.

114. Ibid., p. 8. It is possible that John was the adopted son of either William or Margaret, or both.

115. *Johannes de Mirfeld*, pp. 13–14. On the hospital in general, see *Cartulary of St. Bartholomew's Hospital, Founded 1123*, ed. Nellie Kerling (London: Lund Humphries, 1973), pp. 1–9.

116. *Johannes de Mirfeld*, p. 7. The writers suggest John's reputation as a medical author was a barrier to ordination, but as has been shown, many priests were also physicians. Hartley and Aldridge rightly dismiss the suggestion that Mirfield was a canon at the priory. His will lists him as a chaplain (*capellanus*), and he let a room from the priory, perhaps acting as a salaried official (pp. 3–6).

117. *MPME*, pp. 7–8; *MPME/S*, p. 255; *Johannes de Mirfeld*, p. 9.

118. Rawcliffe, "Hospitals," pp. 2–3.

119. For example, *MPME*, p. 422; Huling E. Ussery, *Chaucer's Physician: Medicine and Literature in Fourteenth-Century England*, Tulane Studies in English 19 (New Orleans: Department of English, Tulane University; 1971), p. 69 n. 32.

120. The known surviving books are devotional in nature. *Medieval Libraries of Great Britain; a List of Surviving Books*, 2d ed., ed. N. R. Ker (London: Royal Historical Society, 1964), p. 123; and *Medieval Libraries of Great Britain, a List of Surviving Books, edited by N. R. Ker, Supplement to the Second Edition*, ed. Andrew G. Watson (London: Royal Historical Society, 1987), p. 47.

121. *Corpus of British Medieval Library Catalogues: The Friars' Libraries*, ed. K. W. Humphreys (London: British Library, 1990), pp. 132–38.

122. The volume, which covers nearly three hundred folios, is found in two manuscripts: London, Gray's Inn MS 4, and British Library, Royal MS 7.F.XI. *Johannes de Mirfeld* prints Latin with facing-page translation of the introduction, conclusion, and single chapter on the duties of the physician (pp. 122–63); the titles of the other 174 chapters are listed on p. 164.

123. "Necesse est enim vt medici sint viri litterati aut quod ab eo qui nouit litteras ad minus artem addiscant" (*Johannes de Mirfeld*, p. 122).

124. "Refertur autem de quodam medico cui debebantur xiii libre ad tres annos soluende, qui cum laboraret in extremis et admoneretur vt confiteretur et eukaristiam sumeret, nichil aliud poterant ab eo extrahere nisi xiii libras et tres annos" (ibid., p. 130).

125. "viles femine et presumptuose istud officium sibi vsurpant et abutantur eo, que nec artem nec ingenium habent, vnde propter causam sue stoliditatis errores maximos operantur, quibus egri multociens interficiuntur" (ibid., p. 122).

126. Ibid., pp. 158–59.

127. The entire text survives in two manuscripts from the late fourteenth century. The first, Oxford, Bodleian Library, Pembroke MS 2, was prepared for the Benedictine abbey of Abingdon, near Oxford. It was later owned by Oxford M.D. Richard Bartlatt (or Bartlot, d. 1557 and buried at the Church of St. Bartholomew the Great; perhaps this Bartlatt was a relative of Thomas Berthelet, the Holborn printer, who held properties taken from the priory in 1543 [*Johannes de Mirfeld*, p. 14]), Fellow of All Souls, who was one of the founders of the College of Physicians of London. Bartlett later gave the book to All Souls. This MS contains the text published as *Sinonoma Bartholomei: A Glossary from a Fourteenth-Century Manuscript in the Library of Pembroke College, Oxford*, ed. J. L. G. Mowat (Oxford: Clarendon Press, 1882). The second, British Library, Harley MS 3, was purchased in 1573 by Dr. John Dee from the widow of a certain Mr. Carey (*Johannes de Mirfeld*, p. 167), and was heavily annotated by Dee

himself, who seemed, by my reading, to have been under the impression he was perusing the *De proprietatibus rerum* of Bartholomaeus Anglicus. Dee's annotations reveal an interest in the recipes the text contains. The manuscript has as its flyleaves the first two leaves of another text of the *Breviarium* in an earlier hand. Part of the text, on the signs of death, is found in a mid-fifteenth-century manuscript; London, Lambeth Palace MS 444 (*Johannes de Mirfeld*, pp. 167–68).

128. *Johannes de Mirfeld*, pp. 50–51. These authors give Latin with facing-page translation of the *Breviarium*'s introduction, conclusion, matter on signs of disease, consumption, weights and measures, and several recipes. *John of Mirfield* gives an English translation of part of Mirfield's surgery, silently omitting the medicinal recipes.

129. *Johannes de Mirfeld*, p. 90.

130. I have identified Albucasis, *Surgery*; Alexander of Tralles, *Practica*; Arnald of Villanova, *Regimen of Health*; Averroes, *Colliget*; Avicenna, *Canon*, books 3, 4; Bartholomaeus Anglicus, *De proprietatibus rerum*; Bernard Gordon, *Lilium, Prognostics*; Bruno the Lombard, *Surgery*; Constantine the African, *Viaticum*; Dioscorides, *Simples*; Galen, commentary on Hippocrates's *Aphorisms* and *Regimen of Acute Diseases*; Galen, *De ingenio sanitatis, Megategni*; Gerard of Cremona, *Commentary on the Viaticum*; Gilbertus Anglicus, *Compendium*; Giles of Corbeil, *Urines*; Haly Abbas, *Liber regius*; Hippocrates, *Aphorisms, Regimen of Acute Diseases*; Isaac Judaeus, *Fevers, Urines*; Johannitius, *Isagoge*; John of Damascus, *Commentary on the Aphorisms*; Lanfrank, *Surgery*; John of Gaddesden, *Rosa*; John Serapion, *Practica*; Macer Floridus; Mesue, *Antidotary, Simples*; Nicholas, *Antidotary*; Platearius, *Circa Instans*; Rasis, *Almansor, Antidotarium, Divisions* (Mirfield also called him "Experimentator"); Roger of Salerno, *Surgery*; Roland of Salerno, *Surgery*; Urso, *Aphorisms*; Walter Agilon, *Practica, Urines*. All these texts were known elsewhere in England during John's time. There are scattered references to other writers less well known: Mr. Thomas Anglicus "astronomus" (cf. MPME, p. 332, Thomas Anglicus, Augustinian friar, 15th c.); Fr. John Helme; Mr. Reginaldus de Villa Nova; Mr. Nicholas Tingewick; the Women of Salerno (*mulieres salernitane*); Robert de Vico Nouo; Mr A. de Sutwille; Robert Grosseteste; Nicholas de Polonia. On the last, see William Eamon and Gundolf Keil, " 'Plebs amat empirica': Nicholas of Poland and His Critique of the Medieval Medical Establishment," *Sudhoffs Archiv* 71 (1987): 180–96. Nicholas was a Dominican friar who studied at Montpellier in the latter part of the thirteenth century.

131. Pembroke MS 2, fol. 126.

132. Ibid., fol. 32.

133. Ibid., fol. 30.

134. Ibid., fol. 33.

135. Ibid., fol. 88.

136. Ibid., fol. 90.

137. Ibid., fol. 99v.

138. Ibid., fol. 148v.

139. Ibid., fol. 203v.

140. Ibid., fol. 108.

141. Ibid., fol. 18v.

142. Ibid., fol. 135v.

143. Ibid., fol. 139v.

144. Ibid., fol. 39v.

145. Ibid., fol. 35.

146. Ibid., fol. 204v.

147. Ibid., fol. 1.

148. The work dates in all likelihood from the middle of the tenth century; *Pseudo-Aristotle, The* Secret of Secrets, ed. W. F. Ryan and Charles B. Schmitt (London: The Warburg Institute, 1982), p. 1; also the extremely useful Middle English and French edition, *Secretum Secretorum: Nine English Versions,* ed. M. A. Manzalaoui, Early English Text Society 276 (Oxford: Oxford University Press, 1977), p. ix.

149. Bacon's commentary is found in *Opera hactenus inedita Rogeri Baconi,* ed. R. Steele et al., 16 vols. (Oxford; [1905/9]–1940), p. 5. An excellent study of the impact the *Secretum* had on Bacon is William Eamon, *Science and the Secrets of Nature: Books of Secrets in Medieval and Early Modern Culture* (Princeton, N.J.: Princeton University Press, 1994), pp. 45–53.

150. "Ars medicinalis remedium non habet nisi regimen sanitatis. Est autem ulterior longae vitae extensio possibilis . . . regimen sanitatis debeat esse in cibo et potu, somno et vigilia, motu et quiete, evacuatione et retentione, aeris dispositione, et passionibus animi" (*The Opus majus of Roger Bacon,* ed. John Henry Bridges, 2 vols., [Oxford, 1897; suppl vol., London, Oxford, and Edinburgh, 1900], 2:204). See also L. J. Rather, " 'The Six Things Non-Natural': A Note on the Origins and Fate of a Doctrine and a Phrase," *Clio Medica* 3 (1968): 337–47; Shulamith Shahar, "The Old Body in Medieval Culture," in *Framing Medieval Bodies,* ed. Sarah Kay and Miri Rubin (Manchester: Manchester University Press, 1994), pp. 160–86.

151. For numerous citations from the *Policraticus* about the good ruler and the nature of his advisers, see Hans Liebeschütz, *Medieval Humanism in the Life and Writings of John of Salisbury* (London: The Warburg Institute, 1950), pp. 23–74. The Book of Deuteronomy warns against imitating the "abominable customs of those other nations" (18:9), and in general outlines an ideal of a moderate ruler, surrounded by adviser priests, who "shall have no holding or patrimony in Israel . . . the Lord is their patrimony" (18:1–2).

152. The humanist textual tradition in which Bacon was working is examined with brilliant insight by James J. Bono, *The Word of God and the Languages of Man: Interpreting Nature in Early Modern Science and Medicine,* vol. 1, *Ficino to Descartes* (Madison: University of Wisconsin Press, 1995).

153.

Et praecipue haec sapientia mundo concessa est per primos, scilicet per Adam et filios ejus, qui receperunt ab ipso Deo specialem congnitionem in hac parte, quatenus vitam suam longius protenderent. Sic videndum est per Aristotelem in libro Secretorum, ubi dicit quod Deus excelsus et gloriosus ordinavit modum et remedium ad temperantiam humorum et conservationem sanitatis, et ad plura adquirenda scilicet ad obviandum passionibus senectutis et ad retardandum eas, et mitigandum hujusmodi; et revalavit ea sanctis et prophetis suis, et quibusdam aliis, sicut patriarchis. (Bacon, *Opus majus,* 2:208).

154. Bacon's disgust for translation of any sort permeates his work. See S. A. Hirsch, "Roger Bacon and Philology," in *Roger Bacon Essays,* ed. A. G. Little (Oxford: Clarendon Press, 1914), pp. 101–51.

155. This study limits itself to examining major writings whose authenticity is reasonably established in internal evidence. It is also not a study of Bacon's sources, most of which are noted in E. Withington's useful "Roger Bacon and Medicine," in *Roger Bacon Essays*, ed. A. G. Little (Oxford: Clarendon Press, 1914), pp. 337–58, in the relevant Latin texts found in Roger Bacon, *De retardatione accidentium senectutis cum aliis opusculis de rebus medicinalibus*, ed. A. G. Little and E. Withington (British Society of Franciscan Studies 14 (Oxford, 1928); and in Mary Catherine Welborn, "The Errors of the Doctors According to Friar Roger Bacon of the Minor Order," *Isis* 18 (1932): 26–62.

156. Michela Pereira, "Un tesoro inestimabile: Elixir e 'Prolongatio Vitae' nell'alchimia de '300," *Micrologus: I discorsi dei corpi* 1 (1993): 164–65.

157. On Grosseteste's ideas of the importance of the study of ancient languages to science, and on Bacon's understanding of Grosseteste's ideas of Christian scholarship, see James A. Weisheipl, "Science in the Thirteenth Century," in *The History of the University of Oxford*, vol. 1, *The Early Oxford Schools*, ed. J. I. Catto and T. A. R. Evans (Oxford: Clarendon Press, 1984), pp. 435–69.

158. In Latin in Bacon, *De . . . rebus medicinalibus*, pp. 150–79. For an English translation, see Welborn, "The Errors of the Doctors." Dating to 1260–70 is suggested by Michael R. McVaugh in *Arnaldi de Villanova*, p. 32 n. 1.

159. The *Opus majus* was sent to the papal court in late 1267 or early 1268; *Roger Bacon's Philosophy of Nature: A Critical Edition with English Translation, Introduction, and Notes of* De multiplicatione specierum *and* De speculis comburentibus, ed. David Lindberg (Oxford: Clarendon Press, 1983), p. xxv.

160. Bacon, *Opus majus*, 2:204–5.

161. *City of God* 16.11, in *Basic Writings of Saint Augustine*, vol. 2, ed. Whitney J. Oates (New York: Random House, 1948), p. 255. What follows is an explanation of how man's fall was both spiritual and physical (p. 256). For more on the "systemic" nature of physical ills, see Peter H. Neibyl, "Sennert, Van Helmont, and Medical Ontology," *Bulletin of the History of Medicine* 45 (1971): 115–37.

162. Bacon, *Opus majus*, 2:205.

163. Here and in other passages, Bacon appears to have in mind the Book of Ecclesiasticus, one of the few parts of (apocryphal) Scripture dealing with medicine directly. Moderation in food, drink, and emotions are recommended throughout, while chapter 37 states that "A man's life lasts a number of days" (25–28). The following chapter, verses 1–15, honors the doctor and advises the faithful to use both him and the medicines of the earth, because the Lord has made them both. Petrus Hispanus (Pope John XXI) cited passages from Ecclesiasticus to begin his popular medical text, *Thesaurus pauperum* (Treasury of the poor), which was written perhaps ten years later than Bacon's medical works.

164. Bacon, *Opus majus*, 2:206–7.

165. Ibid., 2:208–9.

166. Printed in Bacon, *De . . . rebus medicinalibus*, pp. 1–83; but in the *Opus majus*, Bacon referred to "auctor istius libri," which would indicate he did not write the work himself (2: 210). For a thorough investigation of the correct authorship of the treatise, see Agostino Paravicini Bagliani, "Il mito della 'prolongatio vitae' e la corte pontificia del duecento: il 'De retardatione accidentium senectutis,' " in *Medicina e scienze della natura*, pp. 283–326.

167. That is, it had the greatest possible moderating effect; Bacon, *Opus majus,* 2:210.

168. Aequalitas enim elementorum in corporibus illis excludit corruptionem in aeternum (ibid., 2:212). Augustine, in the *City of God,* also discussed the "incorruptible body which is promised to the saints in the resurrection" (*Basic Writings,* p. 153). Bede's *Historia ecclesiastica* is full of examples of saints whose sanctity was known by the fact that their bodies remained uncorrupt: for example, Queen Ethelthryth, a "perpetual virgin, whose body could not either be purified in her tomb," and Cuthbert, who "after eleven years' burial, was found free of corruption" (*Baedae Opera Historica, with an English Translation* by J. E. King, vol. 2); *Ecclesiastical History of the English Nation,* Loeb Classical Library [Cambridge, Mass.: Harvard University Press, 1963], pp. 102–3, 184–85).

169. The ability to fast over long periods, or not to eat at all was, of course, a sign of sanctity. In general, see Caroline Walker Bynum, *Holy Feast and Holy Fast: The Religious Significance of Food to Medieval Women* (Berkeley: University of California Press, 1987), and Rudolph Bell, *Holy Anorexia* (Chicago: University of Chicago Press, 1985).

170. Bacon, *Opus majus,* 2:212.

171. On the history of Christian obsession with bodily integrity and resurrection, see Caroline Walker Bynum, *The Resurrection of the Body in Western Christianity, 200–1336* (New York: Columbia University Press, 1995), esp. "Fragmentation and Ecstasy: The Thirteenth-Century Context," pp. 318–43, which explores some implications of bodily resurrection and controversies over the Beatific Vision. For pontifical interest in prolongation of life (a pope ruled as long as he could live), see Agostino Paravicini Bagliani, "Ruggero Bacone, Bonifacio VIII, e la teoria della 'Prolongatio Vitae'," in *Medicina e scienze della natura,* pp. 327–61. For an intriguing study of what the author argues is a reaction against philosophical images of the body by fourteenth-century French surgeon Henri de Mondeville, see Marie-Christiane Pouchelle, *The Body and Surgery in the Middle Ages,* trans. Rosemary Morris (New Brunswick, N.J.: Rutgers University Press, 1990).

172. On recipes for food and drink that were intended to restore the temperate complexion, see Terence Scully, "The Sickdish in Early French Recipe Collections," in *Health, Disease and Healing in Medieval Culture,* ed. Sheila Campbell, Bert Hall, and David Klausner (New York: St. Martin's Press, 1992), pp. 132–40.

173. Bacon, *Opus majus,* 2:211.

174. The equation of the duties of the good physician with those of the good priest was a medieval commonplace that Bacon and others played upon often. See Gerhard Fichtner, "Christus als Arzt. Ursprünge und Wirkungen eines Motivs," *Frühmittelalterliche Studien* 16 (1982): 1–18 (excellent bibliography); Ralph Arbesman, "The Concept of 'Christus Medicus' in St. Augustine," *Traditio* 10 (1954): 1–28; Jole Agrimi and Chiara Crisciani, "Medicina del corpo e medicina dell'anima: Note sul sapere del medico fino all'inizio del sec. XIII," *Episteme* 10 (1976): 5–102.

175. TK, cols. 463, 893.

176. The *Invectiva* is by and large a defense of poetry against the false rhetoric of the clamoring physicians, who were after all, Petrarch said, only practitioners of the mechanical arts. Petrarch, *Invectiva contra medicum: Testo latino e volgarizzamento di Ser Domenico Silvestri,* ed. Pier Giorgio Ricci (Rome: Storia e Letteratura, 1950); Siraisi, *Medieval and Early Renaissance Medicine,* pp. 46–47.

177. "Sed longum esset prosequi alios defectus vsque ad 36, et longius eorum ramos protendere, nec sufficio" (Bacon, *De . . . rebus medicinalibus*, p. 153).

178. "Vulgus medicorum non congnoscit suam simplicem medicinam, sed committit se rusticis apothecariis, de quibus constat ipsis medicis, quod non intendunt nisi ipsos decipere" (ibid., p. 150).

179. "Libri enim authentici sunt pleni vocabulis Arabicis, Grecis et Caldeis et Hebreis, ita quod non potest homo scire quid auctores velint dicere, ut patet in locis infinitis, et quia ignorant linguam Grecam et Arabicam et Hebream, a quibus infinita vocabula tracta sunt in libris Latinorum, propter quorum ignorantiam non possunt intelligere medicinam nec operari" (ibid., pp. 153–54); further, "ignoratur naturalis philosophia propter translationis peruersitatem: si vnus dicit Aristotelem sentire hoc, alius dicit ipsum sentire contrarium" (ibid., p. 159).

180. "Auctores eandem medicinam simplicem dicunt purgare contraria, i. e. contrarios humores, ut Haly dicit quod sene purgat coleram rubeam, et Auicenna capitulo de fumo terre quod purgat humores adustos, Latini quod melancoliam" (ibid., p. 151); cf. Augustine, *City of God* (in writing about the Trinity): "Neither are there many wisdoms, but one, in which are untold and infinite treasures of things intellectual" (*Basic Writings*, p. 153).

181. On the religious motivation of Bacon's concern with the meaning of words, see R. W. Southern, *Robert Grosseteste: The Growth of an English Mind in Medieval Europe* (Oxford: Clarendon Press, 1986), pp. 15–19.

182. Bacon, *De . . . rebus medicinalibus*, p. 154.

183. For practical descriptions of how medieval medical practitioners made drugs, see "Preparation of Medicines," in Getz, *Healing and Society*, pp. xxxviii–xli.

184. "7us defectus est in fermentatione medicinarum, quia compositum, ut dicit Auicenna, sine fermentatione non valebit . . . hoc est secretum secretorum quod vulgus medicorum omnino ignorat" (Bacon, *De . . . rebus medicinalibus*, pp. 152–53; further, p. 167). Bacon no doubt had in mind the various fermentations described in the fourth book of Aristotle's *Meteorology.*

185. Ibid., p. 165.

186. Bacon, *De . . . rebus medicinalibus*, pp. 151–52; further, p. 163. Cf. Pliny, *Natural History* 8:28–29 (bk. 29, chap. 20), in which Pliny wrote of how treacle was made of vipers' flesh.

187. Bacon, *De . . . rebus medicinalibus*, p. 160.

188. "Difficilis est experientia in medicina" (ibid., p. 161). Bacon's allusion is probably to Hippocrates' the first aphorism.

189. Ibid., p. 161.

190. After noting the folly of slavish attention to medical treatises written only in Greek, Pliny noted that "there is no law to punish criminal ignorance, no instance of retribution. Physicians acquire their knowledge from our dangers, making experiments at the cost of our lives. Only a physician can commit homicide with complete impunity" (*Natural History* 8:195 [bk. 29, chap. 8]).

191. Cf. Pliny, *Natural History* 8:190/91 (bk. 29, chap. 8), in which the writer noted that Romans had lived for more than six hundred years without physicians, but not without medicine (*sine medicina*).

192. Bacon, *De . . . rebus medicinalibus*, p. 163.

193. The stag was thought to live more than over a thousand years; see "Theoretical Justifications for Pharmaceutical Practices," in Getz, *Healing and Society,* pp. xviii–xxii.

194. Welborn, "The Errors of the Doctors," lists the drugs mentioned in *De erroribus* on pp. 54–61. Bacon listed among his favorite remedies "singing, the sight of human beauty, the touch of young girls, warm aromatic waters" and other soothing restoratives (*De . . . rebus medicinalibus,* p. 178), reminding the reader of King David and Abishag (1 Kings 1:1–4).

195. Bacon, *De . . . rebus medicinalibus,* p. 166.

196. Ibid., pp. 166–67.

197. "Aristoteles enim dicit quod vbi terminatur philosophia naturalis, ibi incipit medicina, et naturalis philosophus habet dare principia vltima sanitatis et infirmitatis" (ibid., p. 158); the passage of Aristotle cited is once again *De sensu* 1.436a. See Diego Gracia, "The Structure of Medical Knowledge in Aristotle's Philosophy," *Sudhoffs Archiv* 62 (1978): 23.

198. Faye Marie Getz, "Medical Education in Later Medieval England," in *The History of Medical Education in Britain,* ed. Vivian Nutton and Roy Porter (Amsterdam: Rodopi, 1995), p. 86.

199. *The Works of Geoffrey Chaucer,* pp. 198–205 (VII. 2821–3446).

200. Derek Pearsall, "Hoccleve's *Regement of Princes*: The Poetics of Royal Self-Representation," *Speculum* 69 (1994): 386–410. For Hoccleve's life and a bibliography of his work, see J. A. Burrow, *Thomas Hoccleve* (Aldershot: Variorum, 1994); also *The Regement of Princes A.D. 1411–12,* ed. F. J. Furnivall, Early English Text Society, e.s., 72 (London: K. Paul, Trench, Trubner, 1897).

201. The poem advised moderation in diet, emotion, and exercise over the use of medical practitioners; *The Minor Poems of John Lydgate,* pt. 2, *Secular Poems,* ed. Henry Noble MacCracken, Early English Text Society, o.s., 192 (1934; reprint, 1961), 703–7. The poem is printed with matching verses from the *Regimen sanitatis salernitanum* in Latin that is its source; "John Lydgate's Dietary," ed. Max Forster, *Anglia* 42 (1918): 176–91.

202. *Secretum,* pp. xxii–xlviii.

203.

Cum antiqui sapientes et famossissimi philosophi in suis scriptis et libris sub figuris et integumentis docuerint et reliquerint ex vino, ex lapidibus preciosis, ex oleis, ex vegetabilibus, ex animalibus, ex metallis et ex medijs mineralibus multas medicinas gloriosas et notabiles confici posse, et presertim quandam preciosissimam medicinam quam aliqui philosophorum matrem et imperatricem medicinarum dixerunt, Alij gloriam inestimabilem eandem nominarunt, Alij vero quintam essentiam, lapidem philosophorum et elixir vite nuncupaverunt eandem, cuius medicine virtus tam efficax et admirabilis existeret quod per eam quecunque infirmitates curabiles curarentur faciliter, vita humana ad suum naturalem prorogaretur terminum, et homo in sanitate et viribus naturalibus tam corporis quam anime, fortitudine membrorum, memorie claritate et ingenij viuacitate ad eundem terminum mirabiliter preservaretur, quecunque eciam vulnera curabilia sine difficultate sanarentur que insuper contra omne genus venenorum foret summa et optima medicina. Sed et plura alia comoda nobis et rei publice regni nostri utilissima per eandem fieri possent veluti metallorum transmutationes in verissimum aurum . . . (In Latin with English translation in D. Geohegan, "A Licence of Henry VI to Practise Alchemy," *Ambix* 6 (1957): 10–17).

204. Thomas Norton's *Ordinal of Alchemy*, ed. J. Reidy, Early English Text Society 272 (London and New York: Oxford University Press, 1975), p. 50. Kymer's treatise has not been identified. On prohibitions against alchemy, see Edgar H. Duncan, "The Literature of Alchemy and Chaucer's Canon's Yeoman's Tale: Framework, Theme, and Characters," *Speculum* 43 (1970): 633–56.

205. Charles Webster, "Alchemical and Paracelsian Medicine," in *Health, Medicine, and Mortality Healing in the Sixteenth Century*, ed. Charles Webster (Cambridge: Cambridge University Press, 1979), noted that "Roger Bacon was the major authority cited by Englishmen as sanctioning the quest for eradication of disease and the prolongation of life by alchemical means" (p. 302). For a Continental parallel to Bacon's medical alchemical thinking, see Pearl Kibre, "Albertus Magnus on Alchemy," in *Albertus Magnus and the Sciences: Commemorative Essays*, ed. J. A. Weisheipl (Toronto: Pontifical Institute of Mediaeval Studies, 1980), pp. 187–202.

206. *MPME*, pp. 134–36; *MPME/S*, p. 265.

207. Bacon, *De . . . rebus medicinalibus*, pp. xi–xiii; Getz, "Faculty of Medicine," pp. 378 n. 17, 395.

208. Bacon, *De . . . rebus medicinalibus*, pp. 103–19.

209. "Sed hic est vnus de 36 defectibus qui sunt apud nos, et hoc est propter defectum librorm, vel quia sapientes occultauerunt hanc partem doctrine vel nescierunt; tamen ego scripsi nomina istorum defectuum alibi et partem huius doctrine, secundum quod didici a sapientibus diuersarum linguarum et literature" (ibid., p. 110). The contents of the two treatises overlap considerably.

210. "Oportet igitur medicinam quamlibet compositam fermentari, quia compositum absque fermentatione non valebit, ut dicit Auicenna in .v.to. Nam propter fermentationem ex pluribus rebus simplicibus fit vna medicina, et ex pluribus qualitatibus fit vna qualitas, stans, operans, adquirens aliam virtutem quam in suis simplicibus existat" (ibid., p. 116).

211. The pharmaceutical system Bacon expounded, and its intellectual context are explained thoroughly and masterfully by Michael R. McVaugh in *Arnaldi de Villanova*, pp. 31–51.

212. "Nam ex vera proportione prouenit veritas, virtus, vel proprietas in composito, que in simplicibus non habetur, sed precipue in proportione radicis et rerum sequentium eius operationem. Nam in hiis duobus consistit proprietas et operatio totius compositi" (Bacon, *De . . . rebus medicinalibus*, p. 113; in more detail, *Arnaldi de Villanova*, p. 39).

213. "Caueant igitur arrogantes et proterui in vanitate studentes ex industria eorum componere medicinam, nisi sciant scientiam componendi, quod est impossibile eos noscere propter defectum illius partis scientie que docet cognoscere res que ad inuicem se expoliant, et hec consideratio est gratia compositi totius" (Bacon, *De . . . rebus medicinalibus*, p. 113).

214. "Et si egritudo, contra quam componimus, est frigida, tunc componenda est medicina in qualitate calida secundum contrarium gradum frigiditatis egritudinis" (ibid., p. 112).

215. "Et quandocunque medicina composita excedit in aliqua qualitate: ideo consideranda est eius qualitas, vtrum debeat esse calida vel frigida vel temperata vel sicca vel humida, vtrum secundum Plinium illud quod soluit debet esse calidum" (ibid., pp. 111–12). For the Galenic system, *Arnaldi de Villanova*, pp. 4–8.

216. Cf. *De erroribus*, Bacon, *De . . . rebus medicinalibus*, p. 150.

217. "Nam sicut planta ex suis radicibus, ita compositum ex sua radice vel radicibus sustentatur" (Bacon, *De . . . rebus medicinalibus*, p. 106; also *Arnaldi de Villanova*, pp. 39–45).

218. For a *iera pigra* recipe written by an Englishman contemporary with Bacon, see Gilbertus, *Compendium*, fol. 237; or Getz, *Healing and Society*, p. 222.

219. Bacon, *De . . . rebus medicinalibus*, p. 107.

220. Purgation of peccant humors was discussed frequently in *De erroribus*, for example; ibid., p. 150.

221. "Nam virtutibus confortatis inimicum expellit per sensibilem vel per occultam expulsionem, sicut composita facit medicina que est de genere venenorum" (ibid., p. 105).

222. For vipers' flesh, see esp. ibid., p. 110; for treacle, p. 119; for both together, p. 108; for scriptural, medical, and natural historical contexts, see Jerry Stannard, "Natural History," in *Science in the Middle Ages*, ed. David C. Lindberg (Chicago: University of Chicago Press, 1978), p. 442. Cf. Pliny, *Natural History*: "Theriace vocatur excogitata compositio. Fit ex rebus sexcentis, cum tot remedia dederit natura quae singula sufficerent. Mithridatium antidotum ex rebus LIIII componitur, inter nullas pondere aequali et quarundam rerum sexagesima denarii unius imperata, quo deorum, per Fidem, ista monstrante!" (8:198 [bk. 29, chap. 8]). Pliny continued that the physicians, ignorant of the correct names of drugs, had promoted practices that "ruined the morals of the Empire" (8:199).

223. Linda E. Voigts and Robert P. Hudson, " 'A drynke that men callen dwale to make a man to slepe whyle men kerven him': A Surgical Anesthetic from Late Medieval England," in *Health, Disease and Healing*, ed. Sheila Campbell, Bert Hall, and David Klausner (New York: St. Martin's Press, 1992), pp. 34–56.

224. Known to medical writers as a "stupefacative"; Gilbertus, *Compendium*, fol. 131v; Getz, *Healing and Society*, p. 38.

225. "Et quandocunque intentio nostra est ut medicina quam componimus agat in membro longinquo, et timemus ne digestio prima et secunda frangat virtutem eius, tunc associamus ei medicinam que eam conseruet; et non timemus audaciam duarum digestionum, ymmo ducit eam sanam ad membrum ad quod intendimus, sicut ponimus opium in medicinis tyriace, ut dicit Auicenna in 5o canone" (Bacon, *De . . . rebus medicinalibus*, p. 111). Cf. Gilbertus, *Compendium*, fol. 266 (Getz, *Healing and Society*, p. 247), in which opium was recommended to bring medicine to the kidneys.

226. Bacon, *Opus majus*, 2:204.

227. "Tamen in hiis duobus moderni peccant, in dosi narcoticorum et laxatiuorum, quia quanta est differentia inter calorem naturalem et corpora antiquorum et modernorum, tanta est differentia in dosi scripta in libris antiquis codicis et in illa que debet hodie hominibus exhiberi" (Bacon, *De . . . rebus medicinalibus*, p. 108).

228. Medieval medical texts are full of "rich man, poor man" suggestions for treatment, suiting the drug to the social station of the patient; Gilbertus, *Compendium*, fol. 236v; Getz, *Healing and Society*, pp. 219–20. Likewise, various organs had "social status," the heart being the noblest and requiring the most expensive medicines. Bacon advised compounding medicines that "comforted" especially the heart; *De . . . rebus medicinalibus*, p. 109.

229. A revisionist survey of fifteenth-century literature is David Lawton, "Dullness and the Fifteenth Century," *English Literary History* 54 (1987): 761–99. See also Pear-

sall, "Poetics of Royal Self-Representation"; and Larry Scanlon, "The King's Two Voices: Narrative and Power in Hoccleve's *Regement of Princes*," in *Literary Practice and Social Change in Britain, 1380–1530*, ed. Lee Patterson (Berkeley: University of California Press, 1990), pp. 216–47.

230. Kymer's search for patronage was one of the first and most successful of the fifteenth century. He was followed by the Padua-educated John Free, who took his M.D. at Padua some time after 1461 and was probably secretary to John Tiptoft, earl of Worcester; Getz, "Faculty of Medicine," p. 395; and Rosamond J. Mitchell, *John Free: From Bristol to Rome in the Fifteenth Century* (London: Longman, 1955).

231. The collection included medical books; Getz, "Faculty of Medicine," p. 403. See also A. C. De La Mare, "Manuscripts Given to the University of Oxford by Humfrey, Duke of Gloucester," *Bodleian Library Record* 13, 1 (1988): 30–51; 13, 2 (1989): 112–21. For the medical collections, see Vern L. Bullough, "Duke Humphrey and His Medical Collections," *Renaissance News* 14 (1961): 87–91.

232. Explicit on fols. 102–102v. The text survives in London, British Library, Sloane MS 4, fols. 63–104, from the later fifteenth century. The witness is badly copied, with text missing. It is not Kymer's autograph. The table of contents and two chapters are printed in *Liber Niger Scaccarii*, vol. 2, ed. Thomas Hearn (London, 1774), pp. 550–59. The table of contents is also printed in *Early English Meals and Manners*, ed. Frederick J. Furnivall, Early English Text Society, o.s. 32 (1868; reprint, London: N. Trubner, 1904), pp. lxxxii–lxxxiii.

233. Sloane MS 4, chap. 9, fol. 77v.

234. Ibid., chap. 11, fol. 78v.

235. "Nunc illustrissime princeps . . . vestri autem renes et genitalia operis Venerei inmoderata frequencia aliquantulum debilitantur, quod liquiditas et paucitas vestri seminis denunciant" (ibid., chap. 3, fols. 70v–71; *Liber Niger*, p. 553).

236. "Digestionem impedit, esuriem defalcat, siciem generat, humores corrumpit, spiritus depauperat, calorem naturalem infrigidat, virtutes defectat, operaciones prosternit, humidum radicale consumit, membra liquefacit, morbos nepharios procreat, virum effeminat, amorem hereos et zelotipiam product, oblivionem, pigriciem, negligenciam, et vercordiam parit, vitamque abbreviat" (Sloane MS 4, fol. 84v; *Liber Niger*, p. 557).

237. For the organization of this quasi-legal and educational body, see chapter 4.

Chapter IV
The Institutional and Legal Faces of English Medicine

1. Paul Oskar Kristeller, "The School of Salerno: Its Development and Its Contribution to the History of Learning," *Bulletin of the History of Medicine* 17 (1945): 138–94; Herbert Bloch, *Monte Cassino in the Middle Ages*, vol. 1 (Cambridge, Mass.: Harvard University Press, 1986), pp. 98–110, 127–36.

2. John F. Benton, "Trotula, Women's Problems, and the Professionalization of Medicine in the Middle Ages," *Bulletin of the History of Medicine* 59 (1985): 30–53; Monica Green, "Women's Medical Practice and Health Care in Medieval Europe," *Signs* 14 (1989): 434–73; Green, "Obstetrical and Gynecological Texts in Middle English," *Studies in the Age of Chaucer* 14 (1992): 53–88.

3. In general, Nancy G. Siraisi, *Taddeo Alderotti and His Pupils: Two Generations of Italian Medical Learning* (Princeton, N.J.: Princeton University Press, 1981).

4. On Montpellier, see Luke E. Demaitre, *Doctor Bernard de Gordon: Professor and Practitioner* (Toronto: Pontifical Institute of Mediaeval Studies, 1980).

5. The best general survey of medical education at medieval universities is Nancy G. Siraisi, "Medical Education," in her *Medieval and Early Renaissance Medicine: An Introduction to Knowledge and Practice* (Chicago: University of Chicago Press, 1990), pp. 48–77.

6. Pearl Kibre, "Arts and Medicine in the Universities of the Later Middle Ages," in *The Universities in the Late Middle Ages*, ed. Jozef IJsewijn and Jacques Paquet (Louvain: Leuven University Press, 1978), p. 223.

7. Faye Marie Getz, "The Faculty of Medicine before 1500," in *The History of the University of Oxford*, vol. 2, *Late Medieval Oxford*, ed. Jeremy Catto and Ralph Evans (Oxford: Clarendon Press, 1992), p. 382.

8. Fridolf Kudlien, "Medicine as a 'Liberal Art' and the Question of the Physician's Income," *Journal of the History of Medicine* 31 (1976): 448–59.

9. Darrel W. Amundsen and Gary B. Ferngren, "The Early Christian Tradition," in *Caring and Curing: Health and Medicine in the Western Religious Traditions*, ed. Ronald L. Numbers and Darrel W. Amundsen (New York: Macmillan, 1986), pp. 40–64; Owsei Temkin, *Hippocrates in a World of Pagans and Christians* (Baltimore, Md.: The Johns Hopkins University Press, 1991).

10. For medieval glosses on the meaning of this passage, see Gaines Post, Kimon Giocarinis, and Richard Kay, "The Medieval Heritage of a Humanistic Ideal: '*Scientia Donum Dei Est, unde Vendi Non Potest*,' " *Traditio* 11 (1955): 195–234.

11. Damian Riehl Leader, *A History of the University of Cambridge*, vol. 1, *The University to 1546* (Cambridge: Cambridge University Press, 1988), p. 203; Vern L. Bullough, "The Mediaeval Medical School at Cambridge," *Mediaeval Studies* 24 (1962): 161–68.

12. Getz, "Faculty of Medicine," p. 383.

13. Ibid., pp. 383, 385.

14. See especially J. D. North, "Natural Philosophy in Late Medieval Oxford" and "Astronomy and Mathematics," in *The History of the University of Oxford*, vol. 2, *Late Medieval Oxford*, ed. Jeremy Catto and Ralph Evans (Oxford: Clarendon Press, 1992), 65–174; and Leader, *Cambridge*, p. 204.

15. *The Canterbury Tales, General Prologue*, in *The Works of Geoffrey Chaucer*, ed. F. N. Robinson, 2d ed. (Boston: Houghton Mifflin, 1957), p. 21 (1.434).

16. Pearl Kibre, "Lewis of Caerleon, Doctor of Medicine, Astronomer, and Mathematician (d. 1494?)," *Isis* 43 (1952): 100–108; Getz, "Faculty of Medicine," p. 402 n. 109; C. H. Talbot, "Simon Bredon (c. 1300–1372): Physician, Mathematician and Astronomer," *British Journal for the History of Science* 1 (1962–63): 19–30.

17. Avicenna, *Canon medicinae*, bk. 1, treatise 1.1, translated in *A Source Book in Medieval Science*, ed. Edward Grant (Cambridge, Mass.: Harvard University Press, 1974), pp. 715–16; see also *Saint Thomas Aquinas, The Division and Methods of the Sciences: Questions V and VI of His Commentary on the* De Trinitate *of Boethius*, 3d ed., trans. Armand Maurer (Toronto: Pontifical Institute of Mediaeval Studies, 1963), pp. 13–14 (question 5, article 1, reply to 4).

18. Leader, *Cambridge*, p. 203.

19. London, Wellcome Institute Library, MS 547, fol. 105v, col. 2: "Medicus est artifex sensibilis." See also Faye Marie Getz, "Charity, Translation, and the Language of Medical Learning in Medieval England," *Bulletin of the History of Medicine* 64 (1990): 15.

20. On boys' and girls' education before and outside the university, see Nicholas Orme, *English Schools in the Middle Ages* (London: Methuen, 1973), and Orme, *Education and Society in Medieval and Renaissance England* (London: The Hambledon Press, 1989).

21. James A. Weisheipl, "Curriculum of the Faculty of Arts at Oxford in the Early Fourteenth Century," *Mediaeval Studies* 26 (1964): 143–85, is a clear study of the undergraduate's experience at universities modeled after Paris. See also Leader, *Cambridge*, and North, "Natural Philosophy."

22. Leader, *Cambridge*, p. 203.

23. Getz, "Faculty of Medicine," p. 382.

24. Ibid.

25. Vern L. Bullough has noted of Oxford that many students seem to have studied medicine without taking a degree; "Medical Study at Mediaeval Oxford," *Speculum* 36 (1961): 603–5.

26. *MPME*, pp. 53–54; *MPME/S*, p. 258.

27. *MPME*, pp. 195–96; *MPME/S*, p. 268.

28. Getz, "Faculty of Medicine," p. 383; Leader, *Cambridge*, p. 203.

29. Getz, "Faculty of Medicine," pp. 381–82.

30. Leader, *Cambridge*, p. 202.

31. For Cambridge's medical curriculum, see Leader, *Cambridge*, p. 203.

32. Getz, "Faculty of Medicine," pp. 383–84.

33. Ibid., p. 384.

34. *Rotuli parliamentorum*, vol. 4 (London, n.d.), p. 158.

35. Pearl Kibre, "The Faculty of Medicine at Paris, Charlatanism and Unlicensed Medical Practice in the Later Middle Ages," *Bulletin of the History of Medicine* 27 (1953): 1–20.

36. English physicians may have been impressed by Continental models as well. In Florence, for instance, during the 1380s, educated Florentine physicians created a college of doctors within the already established Guild of Doctors, Apothecaries, and Grocers; Katharine Park, *Doctors and Medicine in Early Renaissance Florence* (Princeton, N.J.: Princeton University Press, 1985), pp. 237–39.

37. *Calendar of Letter-Books Preserved among the Archives of the Corporation of the City of London: Letter-Book K*, ed. R. R. Sharpe (London, 1911), p. 11.

38. Michael T. Walton, "The Advisory Jury and Malpractice in 15th Century London: The Case of William Forest," *Journal of the History of Medicine* 40 (1985): 478–82.

39. In general for the early Tudor period, see Francis Maddison, Margaret Pelling, and Charles Webster, *Essays on the Life and Work of Thomas Linacre* (Oxford: Clarendon Press, 1977); for the Stuart period, Harold J. Cook, *The Decline of the Old Medical Regime in Stuart London* (Ithaca, N.Y., Cornell University Press, 1986).

40. For a study of the difficulty foreigners could have practicing medicine in London, see Harold J. Cook, *Trials of an Ordinary Doctor: Joannes Groenevelt in Seventeenth-Century London* (Baltimore, Md.: The Johns Hopkins University Press, 1994).

41. One clear survey of these developments is Bryce Lyon, *A Constitutional and Legal History of Medieval England* (New York: Harper and Row, 1960).

42. An interesting example is Madeleine Pelner Cosman, "Medieval Medical Malpractice: The Dicta and the Dockets," *Bulletin of the New York Academy of Medicine*, 2d ser., 49 (1973): 22–47.

43. Getz, "Faculty of Medicine," p. 384; by comparison, see the advanced level of cooperation between learned and crafts-based medical practitioners explored in Park, *Doctors and Medicine in Early Renaissance Florence*.

44. In general, see Darrel W. Amundsen, "Medieval Canon Law on Medical and Surgical Practice by the Clergy," *Bulletin of the History of Medicine* 52 (1978): 22–44; and Amundsen, "History of Medical Ethics: Medieval Europe: Fourth to Sixteenth Century," in *The Encyclopedia of Bioethics*, ed. Warren T. Reich, vol. 3 (New York: The Free Press, 1978), pp. 938–51.

45. *The Mirror of Justices*, ed. William Joseph Whittaker, Selden Society 7 (London: B. Quaritch, 1895), p. 137. This passage is followed by one on what to do if a judge performs a false judgment resulting in the death of the defendant.

46. London, Corporation of London Records Office, Miscellaneous Roll CC, membrane 17 dorse. Briefly examined in the *Calendar of Early Mayor's Court Rolls Preserved among the Archives of the Corporation of The City of London at the Guildhall A.D. 1298–1307*, ed. A. H. Thomas (Cambridge: Cambridge University Press, 1924), dated incorrectly as 1321 (p. viii). There is a handwritten calendar of the roll with an index in the Corporation Records Office.

47. The case is mentioned by S. F. C. Milsom, "Reason in the Development of the Common Law," *Law Quarterly Review* 81 (Oct. 1965): 506 n. 20. Milsom suggests that John was perhaps attempting to collect money Alice had refused to pay him.

48. Numerous examples in *Select Cases of Trespass from the King's Courts, 1307–1399*, vols. 1 and 2, ed. Morris S. Arnold, Selden Society 100, 103 (London, 1985, 1987). See esp. 1; lxiv–lxv and 2; 422–23, 425–27. On the murky distinctions regarding *assumpsit* and breach of covenant in medical contexts, see William M. McGovern, Jr., "The Enforcement of Informal Contracts in the Later Middle Ages," *California Law Review* 59 (1971): 1145–93, esp. pp. 1151, 1154, 1170.

49. For the duties of the medieval English coroner in general, see R. F. Hunnisett, *The Medieval Coroner* (Cambridge: Cambridge University Press, 1961). For London, see William Kellaway, "The Coroner in Medieval London," in *Studies in London History Presented to Philip Edmund Jones*, ed. A. E. J. Hollaender and William Kellaway (London: Hodder and Stoughton, 1969), pp. 75–91.

50. *Mirror of Justices*, pp. 29–32. On medieval attitudes to sodomy in general, see John Boswell, *Christianity, Social Tolerance, and Homosexuality: Gay People in Western Europe from the Beginning of the Christian Era to the Fourteenth Century* (Chicago: University of Chicago Press, 1980).

51. *Fleta*, vol. 2, ed. H. G. Richardson and G. O. Sayles, Selden Society 72 (London: B. Quaritch, 1955), p. 65.

52. *Calendar of Coroners' Rolls of the City of London A.D. 1300–1378*, ed. Reginald R. Sharpe (London: Richard Clay and Sons, 1913), pp. 68–69.

53. She meant they had sex with chickens. Matters escalated and involved more people over several days; ibid., pp. 28–30.

54. Ibid., pp. 231–32.

55. Ibid., pp. 12–13.

56. Ibid., pp. 194–95.

57. *Select Cases from the Coroners' Rolls A.D. 1265–1413*, ed. Charles Gross, Selden Society 9 (London: B. Quaritch, 1896), p. 51.

58. *Calendar of Coroners' Rolls of the City of London*, p. 221.

59. On children's lives in general, see Barbara A. Hanawalt, *Growing up in Medieval London: The Experience of Childhood in History* (New York: Oxford University Press, 1993).

60. *Select Cases from the Coroners' Rolls*, p. 8.

61. Ibid., p. 11.

62. *Year Books of Edward II*, vol. 5, *The Eyre of Kent 6&7 Edward II, A.D. 1313–1314*, vol. 1, ed. Frederic William Maitland, Leveson William Vernon Harcourt, and William Craddock Bolland. Selden Society 24 (London: B. Quaritch, 1910), p. 87.

63. *Calendar of Coroners' Rolls of the City of London*, pp. 170–71.

64. See Barbara A. Kellum, "Infanticide in England in the Later Middle Ages," *History of Childhood Quarterly* 1 (1973–74): 367–88; R. H. Helmholz, "Infanticide in the Province of Canterbury during the Fifteenth Century," *History of Childhood Quarterly* 2 (1974–75): 379–90; and the excellent study, Zefira Entin Rokéah, "Unnatural Child Death among Christians and Jews in Medieval England," *Journal of Psychohistory* 18 (1990–91): 181–226.

65. *Rolls of the Justices in Eyre being the Rolls of Pleas and Assizes for Yorkshire in 3 Henry III (1218–19)*, ed. Doris Mary Stenton, Selden Society 56 (London: B. Quaritch, 1937), pp. 248 ff.

66. *Calendar of Coroners' Rolls of the City of London*, p. 61.

67. Ibid., pp. 219–20.

68. Ibid., pp. 43–44.

69. Ibid., pp. 167–68.

70. *Select Cases from the Coroners' Rolls*, p. 21.

71. *Borough Customs*, vol. 1, ed. Mary Bateson, Selden Society 18 (London: B. Quaritch, 1904), p. 30.

72. *Introduction to the Curia Regis Rolls, 1199–1230*, ed. C. T. Flower, Selden Society 62 (London: B. Quaritch, 1944), pp. 380–87.

73. *Calendar of Coroners' Rolls of the City of London*, pp. 3–4; *MPME*, p. 377.

74. *Select Cases in the Court of King's Bench under Edward I*, vol. 1, ed. G. O. Sayles, Selden Society 55 (London: B. Quaritch, 1936), pp. 120–28, surgeon on p. 126. The importance of prognosis is highlighted here, which is probably the reason recognized surgeons were summoned.

75. *Calendar of Early Mayor's Court Rolls*, p. 51. It is possible that the court believed the man was practicing magic.

76. *The Annals of the Barber-Surgeons of London*, ed. Sidney Young (London: Blades, Tast and Blades, 1890), p. 25.

77. *Memorials of London and London Life*, ed. Henry T. Riley (London: Longman, 1868), pp. 274, 337.

78. For a medieval description of epilepsy, see Faye Marie Getz, *Healing and Society in Medieval England: A Middle English Translation of the Pharmaceutical Writings of Gilbertus Anglicus* (Madison: University of Wisconsin Press, 1991), pp. 20–27.

79. *Calendar of Coroners' Rolls of the City of London*, pp. 5–6.

80. *Select Cases from the Coroners' Rolls*, pp. 5–6.

81. *Rolls of the Justices in Eyre being the Rolls of Pleas and Assizes for Gloucestershire, Warwickshire, and Staffordshire, 1221, 1222*, ed. Doris Mary Stenton, Selden Society 59 (London: B. Quaritch, 1940), p. 108.

82. *Select Cases from the Coroners' Rolls*, p. 17.

83. *Calendar of Coroners' Rolls of the City of London*, pp. 22–23; for quinsy (peritonsillar abscess), see Getz, *Healing and Society*, pp. 101–5.

84. *Select Cases from the Coroners' Rolls*, p. 62.

85. Ibid., pp. 4–5.

86. Ibid., pp. 68–69.

87. *Calendar of Coroners' Rolls of the City of London*, pp. 198–99.

88. Ibid., pp. 23–24.

89. Ibid., pp. 11–12.

90. *Select Cases in Chancery A.D. 1364 to 1471*, ed. William Paley Baildon, Selden Society 10 (London: B. Quaritch, 1896), p. xliii; Getz, *Healing and Society*, pp. 51–54.

91. *Select Cases Concerning the Law Merchant A.D. 1270–1638*, vol 1, *Local Courts*, ed. Charles Gross, Selden Society 23 (London: B. Quaritch, 1908), p. 36.

92. *Select Cases in the Court of King's Bench under Edward I*, vol. 3, ed. G. O. Sayles, Selden Society 58 (London: B. Quaritch, 1939), p. 31. From about 1215, English ecclesiastical courts used juries of women to examine husbands alleged to be impotent: Jacqueline Murray, "On the Origins and Role of 'Wise Women' in Causes for Annulment on the Grounds of Male Impotence," *Journal of Medieval History* 16 (1990): 235–49.

93. *Calendar of Coroners' Rolls of the City of London*, pp. 24–25.

94. *Select Cases in the Court of King's Bench under Richard II, Henry IV, and Henry V*, ed. G. O. Sayles, Selden Society 88 (London: B. Quaritch, 1971), p. 63; the mixture of Anglo-Norman and Latin is typical in such documents.

95. *The London Eyre of 1276*, ed. Martin Weinbaum (Leicester: London Records Society, 1976), pp. 72–73.

96. *Select Cases from the Coroners' Rolls*, p. 79.

97. *Calendar of Coroners' Rolls of the City of London*, pp. 53–54. Prisoners were expected to provide their own food and water.

98. Ibid., pp. 139–40. On care of the elderly, especially peasants in rural areas, see Elaine Clark, "Some Aspects of Social Security in Medieval England," *Journal of Family History* 7 (1982): 307–20; on legal concepts of who was considered elderly, see Shulamith Shahar, "Who Were Old in the Middle Ages," *Social History of Medicine* 6 (1993): 313–41.

99. In general, Jean-Claude Schmitt, "Le suicide au moyen âge," *Annales E. S. C.* 31 (1976): 3–28; also Michael MacDonald and Terence R. Murphy, *Sleepless Souls: Suicide in Early Modern England* (Oxford: Clarendon Press, 1990), esp. "Suicide in the Middle Ages," pp. 16–23.

100. *Calendar of Coroners' Rolls of the City of London*, pp. 36–37; on frenzy, see Getz, *Healing and Society*, pp. 10–13.

101. *Select Cases from the Coroners' Rolls*, p. 49.

102. *Year Books of Edward II: The Eyre of London 14 Edward II, A.D. 1321*, vol. 1, ed. Helen M. Cam, Selden Society 85 (London: B. Quaritch, 1968), p. 93.

103. *Calendar of Coroners' Rolls of the City of London*, p. 249.

104. Ibid., pp. 60–61.

105. *The Roll of the Shropshire Eyre of 1256*, ed. Alan Harding, Selden Society 96 (London, 1981), p. 276.

106. *Rolls of the Justices in Eyre, . . . Yorkshire*, p. 248.

107. *Fleta*, p. 89.

108. *Mirror of Justices*, p. 139.

109. Ibid., p. 138.

110. *Select Pleas of the Crown, vol. 1 A.D. 1200–1225*, ed. F. W. Maitland, Selden Society 1 (London: B. Quaritch, 1888), pp. 66–67.

111. Ibid., p. 119.

112. *Select Cases in the Court of King's Bench under Edward I*, 3; 66.

113. *Borough Customs*, vol. 2, ed. Mary Bateson, Selden Society 21 (London: B. Quaritch, 1906), p. 150.

114. Ibid., pp. 156–57.

115. *Select Cases in the Court of King's Bench under Edward III*, vol. 4, ed. G. O. Sayles, Selden Society 82 (London: B. Quaritch, 1965), p. 163. In this and in similar cases, the court seemed to regard the malefactor as eccentric rather than dangerous.

116. Ibid., pp. 42–43.

117. On leprosy in England, see Nicholas Orme and Margaret Webster, "Leprosy and Its Consequences," in *The English Hospital, 1070–1570* (New Haven, Conn.: Yale University Press, 1995), pp. 23–31; on medieval understanding of the meaning of the disease, see Saul Nathaniel Brody, *The Disease of the Soul: Leprosy in Medieval Literature* (Ithaca, N.Y.: Cornell University Press, 1974); Peter Richards, *The Medieval Leper and His Northern Heirs* (Cambridge, England: D. S. Brewer, 1977).

118. *Calendar of Select Pleas and Memoranda of the City of London*, vol. 3, ed. A. H. Thomas (Cambridge: Cambridge University Press, 1926), p. 289.

119. *Select Cases in the Court of King's Bench under Richard II, Henry IV, and Henry V*, pp. 45–46.

120. *Select Cases Concerning the Law Merchant*, vol. 1, p. 14.

121. *Leet Jurisdiction in the City of Norwich during the xiiith and xivth Centuries*, ed. William Hudson, Selden Society 5 (London: B. Quaritch, 1892), p. 68.

122. *Select Cases in the Court of King's Bench under Richard II, Henry IV, and Henry V*, p. 247.

123. *Select Cases in the Court of King's Bench under Edward I*, vol. 3, p. c.

124. Philip Ziegler, *The Black Death* (London: Collins, 1969); Faye Marie Getz, "Black Death and the Silver Lining: Meaning, Continuity, and Revolutionary Change in Histories of Medieval Plague," *Journal of the History of Biology* 24 (1991): 265–89; for primary sources on all of Europe, *The Black Death*, ed. and trans. Rosemary Horrox (Manchester: Manchester University Press, 1994).

125. *Public Works in Mediaeval Law,* vol. 1, ed. C. T. Flower, Selden Society 32 (London: B. Quaritch, 1915), p. 269. In rural areas especially, the upkeep of roads and ditches was considered the responsibility of local property owners. When facilities were not kept up, the law usually tried to determine who had performed upkeep last in order to decide who should do it in the future.

126. *Public Works in Mediaeval Law,* vol. 2, ed. C. T. Flower, Selden Society 40 (London: B. Quaritch, 1923), pp. 88–89.

127. *Select Cases in the Court of King's Bench under Richard II, Henry IV, and Henry V,* p. xxii.

128. *Select Cases in the Court of King's Bench under Edward III,* 4; 110–11. For similar cases, leading up to a popular uprising against wage controls that were a reaction to labor shortages, see *The Peasants' Revolt of 1381,* ed. R. B. Dobson (London: Macmillan, 1970).

129. *Calendar of Coroners' Rolls of the City of London,* p. 1.

130. Ibid., pp. 116–17.

131. *Rolls of the Justices in Eyre, . . . Yorkshire,* p. 378.

132. *Calendar of Coroners' Rolls of the City of London,* pp. 33–34.

133. *Year Books of Edward II,* vol 5, p. 111. For learned commentary on this remarkably persistent notion, see the landmark study by Joan Cadden, *Meanings of Sex Difference in the Middle Ages: Medicine, Science, and Culture* (Cambridge: Cambridge University Press, 1993), pp. 93–97.

134. *Select Cases in the Court of King's Bench under Edward I,* 3:31.

135. *Fleta,* p. 31; for more information on similar cases, see Thomas R. Forbes, "A Jury of Matrons," *Medical History* 32 (1988): 23–33.

136. *Fleta,* pp. 60–61.

137. *Select Cases in the Court of King's Bench under Edward I,* vol. 2, ed. G. O. Sayles, Selden Society 57 (London: B. Quaritch, 1938), pp. 151–53.

138. *Leet Jurisdiction in the City of Norwich,* p. 70. The barber was performing a typical function of his craft: bloodletting.

139. For England and France, see Vern L. Bullough, "Training of the Nonuniversity-Educated Medical Practitioners in the Later Middle Ages," *Journal of the History of Medicine* 14 (1959): 446–58.

140. For York, see G. A. Auden, "The Gild of Barber Surgeons of the City of York," *Proceedings of the Royal Society of Medicine* 21, 2 (1928): 1400–1406; and Margaret C. Barnet, "The Barber-Surgeons of York," *Medical History* 12 (1968): 19–30. For late medieval English surgery in general, see Carole Rawcliffe, "The Surgeons," in *Medicine and Society in Later Medieval England* (Stroud: Alan Sutton, 1995), pp. 125–47. For London, see *The Annals of the Barber-Surgeons;* John Flint South, *Memorials of the Craft of Surgery in England,* ed. D'Arcy Power (London: Cassell and Co., 1886); for useful primary source material but not interpretation, see *The Cutting Edge: Early History of the Surgeons of London,* ed. R. Theodore Beck (London: Lund Humphries, 1974); and Jessie Dobson and R. Milnes Walker, *Barbers and Barber-Surgeons of London: A History of the Barbers' and Barber-Surgeons' Companies* (Oxford: Blackwell Scientific Publications, 1979).

141. Heather Swanson, "The Illusion of Economic Structure: Craft Guilds in Late Medieval English Towns," *Past and Present* no. 121 (1988): 29–48.

142. Judith M. Bennett, "Medieval Women, Modern Women: Across the Great Divide," in *Culture and History, 1350–1600: Essays on English Communities, Identities and Writing*, ed. David Aers (London: Harvester Wheatsheaf, 1992), pp. 147–75.

143. Martha Carlin, *Medieval Southwark* (London: The Hambledon Press, 1996), pp. 174–77; Bennett, "Medieval Women," p. 156.

144. R. B. Dobson, "Admissions to the Freedom of the City of York in the Later Middle Ages," *Economic History Review* 26 (1973): 14 n. 2.

145. South, *Memorials*, pp. 16–19.

Chapter V
Well-Being without Doctors

1. Duke Humfrey's contacts with Italian humanists are examined in detail in Roberto Weiss, *Humanism in England during the Fifteenth Century*, 2d ed. (Oxford: Basil Blackwell, 1957). Weiss adopts the popular assertion that "English humanism begins only after Poggio [Bracciolini] had returned to Italy [in 1422]" (p. 22).

2. On this point, and on medieval humanism in general, see R. W. Southern, *Scholastic Humanism and the Unification of Europe*, vol. 1, *Foundations* (Oxford: Blackwell Publishers, 1995), pp. 17–57.

3. A recent introduction is Charles G. Nauert, Jr., *Humanism and the Culture of Renaissance Europe* (Cambridge: Cambridge University Press, 1995); an introduction to the transmission of classical texts is L. D. Reynolds and N. G. Wilson, *Scribes and Scholars: A Guide to the Transmission of Greek and Latin Literature*, 2d ed. (Oxford: Clarendon Press, 1974); in England, see Joseph M. Levine, *Humanism and History: Origins of Modern English Historiography* (Ithaca, N.Y.: Cornell University Press, 1987); for medicine, see Jerome J. Bylebyl, "Medicine, Philosophy, and Humanism in Renaissance Italy," in *Science and the Arts in the Renaissance*, ed. John W. Shirley and F. David Hoeniger (Washington, D.C.: The Folger Shakespeare Library, 1985), pp. 27–49.

4. On humanism and writing in the vernacular, the *locus classicus* is Dante's work on eloquence in the vernacular: *De vulgari eloquentia*, ed. Airstide Marigo (Florence: Felice Le Monnier, 1948), which has Latin with facing-page translation in Italian; in English translation, *Dante's Treatise "De Vulgari Eloquentia,"* trans. A. G. Ferrers Howell (London: Kegan Paul, 1890). Secondary sources include Clare Carroll, "Humanism and English Literature in the Fifteenth Century," in *The Cambridge Companion to Renaissance Humanism*, ed. Jill Kraye (Cambridge: Cambridge University Press, 1996), pp. 189–202, 246–68. On vernacular translation and composition as a typical interest of humanists, see Pearl Kibre, "The Intellectual Interests Reflected in Libraries of the Fourteenth and Fifteenth Centuries," in *Studies in Medieval Science: Alchemy, Astrology, Mathematics and Medicine* (London: The Hambledon Press, 1984), pp. 257–97, which contains specific examples of vernacular translations in humanist book collections.

5. An excerpt from Daniel's uroscopy is edited with extensive notes and introductory material by Ralph Hanna III, "Henry Daniel's *Liber Uricrisiarum* (Excerpt)," in *Popular and Practical Science of Medieval England*, ed. Lister M. Matheson (East Lansing, Mich.: Colleagues Press, 1994), pp. 185–218. The treatise, but not the prologue, was first edited by Joanne Jasin as *A Critical Edition of the Middle English* Liber Uricrisiarum *in Wellcome MS 225* (Ph.D. diss. Tulane University 1983). She has published an article from the edition, "The Transmission of Learned Medical Literature in the Middle

English *Liber Uricrisiarum*," *Medical History* 37 (1993): 313–29. She is preparing an edition of the text for publication.

6. The uroscopy itself is in English but the prologue, reflecting on the importance of vernacular translation, is in Latin. Daniel, like Dante, apparently, preferred to address his more theoretical musings to fellow readers of Latin and conceal them somewhat from readers of the vernacular.

7. London, British Library, Royal MS 17D, fol. 1v, cited in Faye Marie Getz, "Charity, Translation, and the Language of Medical Learning in Medieval England," *Bulletin of the History of Medicine* 64 (1990): 13; for an overview of Middle English vernacular medical texts, see Linda E. Voigts, "Multitudes of Middle English Medical Manuscripts, or the Englishing of Science and Medicine," in *Manuscript Sources of Medieval Medicine: A Book of Essays*, ed. Margaret R. Schleissner (New York: Garland Publishing, 1995), pp. 183–95.

8. On the bibliography of rhetoric, see Dominic A. Larusso, "Rhetoric in the Italian Renaissance," in *Renaissance Eloquence: Studies in the Theory and Practice of Renaissance Rhetoric* (Berkeley: University of California Press, 1983), pp. 37–55; James J. Murphy, *Medieval Rhetoric: A Select Bibliography* (Toronto: University of Toronto Press, 1989).

9. William J. Courtenay, "From Schools to Court Circles: Scholasticism and Middle English Literature," in *Schools and Scholars in Fourteenth-Century England* (Princeton, N.J.: Princeton University Press, 1987), pp. 374–80. Courtenay argues that writing in the vernacular in England was connected to philosophical trends away from nominalism and toward realism. A more strictly literary outline of the development of English as a literary language is A. G. Rigg's preface to *Latin Verses in the* Confessio Amantis: *An Annotated Translation*, by John Gower, ed. Sian Echard and Claire Fanger (East Lansing, Mich.: Colleagues Press, 1991), pp. xiii–xxiv.

10. On the spread of English ideas to the Continent and the influence of French and Italian humanistic ideas in England, see Courtenay, "English Ties with Continental Learning," in *Schools and Scholars*, pp. 147–67.

11. See Anne Hudson, *The Premature Reformation: Wycliffite Texts and Lollard History* (Oxford: Clarendon Press, 1988), esp. "The Context of Vernacular Wycliffism," pp. 390–445. On the topic throughout the medieval West, see the essays in *Heresy and Literacy, 1000–1530*, ed. Peter Biller and Anne Hudson (Cambridge: Cambridge University Press, 1994), esp. Hudson, "*Laicus Litteratus*: The Paradox of Lollardy," pp. 222–36.

12. For a chronological summary of Chaucer's travels, see *The Works of Geoffrey Chaucer*, ed. F. N. Robinson, 2d ed. (Boston: Houghton Mifflin Co., 1957), pp. xix–xxviii; for his life in more detail, *Chaucer Life-Records*, ed. Martin M. Crow and Clair C. Olson from materials compiled by John M. Manly and Edith Rickert, with the assistance of Lilian J. Redstone and others (London: Oxford University Press, 1966).

13. Cited in Getz, "Charity," p. 1 n. 2. See also Nancy G. Siraisi, *Medieval and Early Renaissance Medicine: An Introduction to Knowledge and Practice* (Chicago: University of Chicago Press, 1990), pp. 46–47; and Gerhard Baader, "Medizin und Renaissancehumanismus," in *Istoriga dalla Madaschegna: Festschrift für Nikolaus Mani*, ed. Friedrun R. Hau, Gundolf Keil, and Charlotte Schubert (Hannover: Horst Wellm Verlag, 1985), pp. 115–39.

14. Explained in more detail using vernacular sources in English in Faye Marie Getz, *Healing and Society in Medieval England: A Middle English Translation of the Pharma-*

ceutical Writings of Gilbertus Anglicus (Madison: University of Wisconsin Press, 1991), pp. xxx–xli.

15. L. J. Rather, "The 'Six Things Non-Natural': A Note on the Origins and Fate of a Doctrine and a Phrase," *Clio Medica* 3 (1968): 337–47.

16. On the humanistic contempt for those who request payment for learned advice, see Gaines Post, Kimon Giocarinis, and Richard Kay, "The Medieval Heritage of a Humanistic Ideal: '*Scientia Donum Dei Est, unde Vendi Non Potest,*' " *Traditio* 11 (1955): 195–234.

17. *The Works of Geoffrey Chaucer,* p. 199 (VII.2837–39).

18. Ibid., p. 200 (VII.2866–67).

19. Ibid., p. 203 (VII.3257).

20. For an interpretation of this tale as Chaucer's attack on flattery, see Larry Scanlon, "The *Nun's Priest's Tale*: The Authority of Fable," in *Narrative, Authority, and Power: The Medieval Exemplum and the Chaucerian Tradition* (Cambridge: Cambridge University Press, 1994), pp. 229–44.

21. For an astronomical study of the tale, see J. D. North, "The Nun's Priest's Tale," in *Chaucer's Universe* (Oxford: Clarendon Press, 1988), pp. 456–68.

22. *The Works of Geoffrey Chaucer,* p. 149 (VI.459–60).

23. Ibid., p. 21 (I.442–44).

24. Cf. Ecclesiasticus 19:22, 29–31: "The knowledge of wickedness is not wisdom, nor is there good sense in the advice of sinners. . . . Yet you can tell a man by his looks and recognize good sense at first sight. A man's clothes, and the way he laughs, and his gait, reveal his character."

25. *The Works of Geoffrey Chaucer,* p. 23 (I.629–32).

26. For lovesickness and pathology, see Mary Frances Wack, *Lovesickness in the Middle Ages: The* Viaticum *and Its Commentaries* (Philadelphia: University of Pennsylvania Press, 1990).

27. *The Works of Geoffrey Chaucer,* p. 322 (prosa 2).

28. Ibid., p. 322 (prosa 3).

29. The role of the teacher as healer should not be dismissed here as merely "metaphorical." The poet John Gower, mentioned by Chaucer as "moral Gower" at the end of *Troilus and Criseyde* ("O moral Gower, this book I directe/To the"; *The Works of Geoffrey Chaucer,* p. 479 [V.1856–57]), wrote in all three literary languages—English, French, Latin. In his own multilingual poem, *Confessio amantis* (written ca. 1386–93), he described the various philosophies. Under the heading "Rhetoric," he noted that "These three are efficacious: herb, stone, speech;/And yet by force of word's weight more is moved (Herba, lapis, sermo, tria sunt virtute repleta, /Vis tamen ex verbi pondere plura facit)" (*Latin Verses in the* Confessio amantis, ed. Sian Echard and Claire Fanger (East Lansing, Mich.: Colleagues Press, 1991), pp. 78–79. Gower seems to be offering rhetoric as something that has the actual power to heal. On the phrase "herbs, words, stones," see Getz, *Healing and Society,* p. 310 n. 286/4–5.

30. Martha Carlin, "Medieval English Hospitals," in *The Hospital in History,* ed. Lindsay Granshaw and Roy Porter (London and New York: Routledge, 1989), p. 31.

31. Ibid., pp. 21, 25, 33.

32. For legal, popular, and ecclesiastical opinion as to who was old and what this meant, see Shulamith Shahar, "Who Were Old in the Middle Ages," *Social History of Medicine* 6 (1993): 313–41; for care of the elderly outside hospitals, especially of peas-

ants in rural areas, see Elaine Clark, "Some Aspects of Social Security in Medieval England," *Journal of Family History* 7 (1982): 307–20.

33. Carole Rawcliffe, "The Hospitals of Later Medieval London," *Medical History* 28 (1984): 11.

34. Rawcliffe, "Hospitals," pp. 11–12. Rawcliffe describes the regimen of prayer at one London hospital as a "treadmill of pious gratitude" (p. 12).

35. Nicholas Orme and Margaret Webster, *The English Hospital, 1070–1570* (New Haven, Conn.: Yale University Press, 1995), p. 15.

36. Ibid., p. 20.

37. Ibid., p. 35.

38. On arrangements for medical care within monastic houses in England, see Stanley Rubin, "The Monastic Infirmary," in *Medieval English Medicine* (New York: Barnes and Noble, 1974), pp. 172–88.

39. Orme and Webster, *Hospital*, p. 23.

40. Carlin,"Hospitals," p. 32.

41. Rawcliffe, "Hospitals," p. 12.

42. Orme and Webster, *Hospital*, pp. 72–74. For an excellent description of the day-to-day management of a medieval English hospital through several hundred years, see Martha Carlin, *Medieval Southwark* (London: The Hambledon Press, 1996), pp. 75–85; for hospitals around Cambridge, see Miri Rubin, "Development and Change in English Hospitals, 1100–1500," in *The Hospital in History*, ed. Lindsay Granshaw and Roy Porter (London: Routledge, 1989), pp. 41–59, which concentrates on hospitals as systems of poor relief; more generally, Rubin, *Charity and Community in Medieval Cambridge* (Cambridge: Cambridge University Press, 1987).

43. In general, David Loschky and Ben D. Childers, "Early English Mortality," *Journal of Interdisciplinary History* 24 (1993): 85–97. On famine, see William Chester Jordan, *The Great Famine: Northern Europe in the Early Fourteenth Century* (Princeton, N.J.: Princeton University Press, 1996); Ian Kershaw, "The Great Famine and Agrarian Crisis in England, 1315–1322," *Past and Present* no. 59 (1973): 3–50. On plague, Mark Bailey, "Demographic Decline in Late Medieval England: Some Thoughts on Recent Research," *Economic History Review* 49 (1996): 1–19; John Hatcher, *Plague, Population and the English Economy, 1348–1530* (London: Macmillan, 1977).

44. Rawcliffe, "Hospitals," p. 11.

45. Ronald C. Finucane, "The Use and Abuse of Medieval Miracles," *History* 60 (1975): 1–10; in more detail in his book *Miracles and Pilgrims: Popular Beliefs in Medieval England* (Totowa, N.J.: Rowman and Littlefield, 1977). For a survey of the literature as well as a thoughtful study especially of the European continent in the earlier Middle Ages, see Patrick J. Geary, *Living with the Dead in the Middle Ages* (Ithaca, N.Y.: Cornell University Press, 1994); also Peter Brown's classic *The Cult of Saints: Its Rise and Function in Latin Christianity* (Chicago: University of Chicago Press, 1981).

46. *The Works of Geoffrey Chaucer*, p. 17 (I.17–18).

47. On the nature of miracles performed and on the variety of suppliants, see Eleanora Gordon, "Child Health in the Middle Ages as Seen in the Miracles of Five English Saints, A.D. 1150–1220," *Bulletin of the History of Medicine* 60 (1986): 502–22; Gordon, "Accidents among Medieval Children as Seen from the Miracles of Six English Saints and Martyrs," *Medical History* 35 (1991): 145–63.

48. For the mechanics of collecting a "library" of relics, and for the important commercial value of such collections to their holders, see Denis Bethell, "The Making of a Twelfth-Century Relic Collection," *Studies in Church History* 8 (1972): 61–72, which explores the relics of Reading Abbey; and Bethell, "The Miracles of St. Ithamar," *Analecta Bollandiana* 89 (1971): 421–37, which describes the fortunes of the body parts of this Anglo-Saxon bishop.

49. On the presence of the personality of the individual in relics, see Katharine Park, "The Life of the Corpse: Division and Dissection in Late Medieval Europe," *Journal of the History of Medicine* 50 (1995): 119.

50. Park, "Life of the Corpse," pp. 111–32.

51. Finucane, "Use and Abuse," p. 7; Finucane also notes a number of arguments between observers about whether a person was alive or dead, some of which lasted for days before the matter was resolved.

Bibliography

Primary Sources

Manuscripts

London, British Library, Harley MS 3.

London, British Library, Royal MS 17D.

London, British Library, Royal MS 7.F.XI.

London, British Library, Sloane MS 4.

London, British Library, Sloane MS 6.

London, Corporation of London Records Office, Miscellaneous Roll CC.

London, Gray's Inn MS 4.

London, Lambeth Palace MS 444.

London, Wellcome Institute Library, MS 547.

Oxford, Bodleian Library, Digby MS 160.

Oxford, Bodleian Library, Pembroke MS 2.

Printed Sources

Alfred of Sareshel. *Alfred of Sareshel's Commentary on the* Metheora *of Aristotle.* Edited by James K. Otte. Leiden: E. J. Brill, 1988.

———. *Alfred of Sareshel (Alfredus Anglicus), De motu cordis.* Edited by Clemens Baeumker. *Beiträge zur Geschichte der Philosophie des Mittelalters* 23 (1923): pts. 1–2.

The Annals of the Barber-Surgeons of London. Edited by Sidney Young. London: Blades, Tast and Blades, 1890.

Aquinas, Thomas. *Saint Thomas Aquinas, The Division and Methods of the Sciences: Questions V and VI of His Commentary on the* De Trinitate *of Boethius.* 3d ed. Translated by Armand Maurer. Toronto: Pontifical Institute of Mediaeval Studies, 1963.

Arnald of Villanova. *Arnaldi de Villanova, Opera Medica Omnia II: Aphorismi de Gradibus.* Edited by Michael R. McVaugh. Granada-Barcelona: Seminarium Historiae Medicae Granatensis, 1975.

Augustine of Hippo. *Basic Writings of Saint Augustine.* Vol. 2. Edited by Whitney J. Oates. New York: Random House, 1948.

Bacon, Roger. *Opera hactenus inedita Rogeri Baconi.* Edited by R. Steele et al. 16 vols. Oxford, [1905/9]–1940.

———. *The Opus majus of Roger Bacon.* Edited by John Henry Bridges. 2 vols. Oxford, 1897. Suppl. vol., London, Oxford, and Edinburgh, 1900.

———. *De retardatione accidentium senectutis cum aliis opusculis de rebus medicinalibus.* Edited by A. G. Little and E. Withington. British Society of Franciscan Studies 14. Oxford, 1928.

———. *Roger Bacon's Philosophy of Nature: A Critical Edition with English Translation, Introduction, and Notes of* De multiplicatione specierum *and* De speculis comburentibus. Edited by David Lindberg. Oxford: Clarendon Press, 1983.

Bartholomaeus Anglicus. *De proprietatibus rerum.* 1601. Reprint, Frankfurt am Main: Minerva G. M. B. H., 1964.

Bartholomaeus Anglicus. *On the Properties of Things: John Trevisa's Translation of* Bartholomaeus Anglicus De Proprietatibus Rerum, *A Critical Text.* Edited by M. C. Seymour et al. 3 vols. Oxford: Clarendon Press, 1975–88.

Bede. *Baedae Opera Historica, with an English Translation* by J. E. King. Vol. 2, *Ecclesiastical History of the English Nation.* Loeb Classical Library. Cambridge, Mass.: Harvard University Press, 1963.

———. *Bedae Venerabilis Opera: Pars VI, Opera Didascalica, 1.* Edited by Charles W. Jones. Corpus Christianorum Series Latina, vol. 123A. Turnoholti: Typographi Brepols, 1975.

———. *Bede's Ecclesiastical History of the English People.* Edited by Bertram Colgrave and R. A. B. Mynors. Oxford: Clarendon Press, 1969.

The Black Death. Edited and translated by Rosemary Horrox. Manchester: Manchester University Press, 1994.

Blund, Johannes. *Tractatus de anima.* Edited by D. A. Callus and R. W. Hunt. London: Oxford University Press, 1970.

Borough Customs. Vol. 1. Edited by Mary Bateson. Selden Society 18. London: B. Quaritch, 1904.

Borough Customs. Vol. 2. Edited by Mary Bateson. Selden Society 18. London: B. Quaritch, 1906.

Calendar of Close Rolls Preserved in the Public Record Office; Edward III, A.D. 1327–1330. London: HMSO, 1896.

Calendar of Coroners' Rolls of the City of London A.D. 1300–1378. Edited by Reginald R. Sharpe. London: Richard Clay and Sons, 1913.

Calendar of Early Mayor's Court Rolls Preserved among the Archives of the Corporation of The City of London at the Guildhall A.D. 1298–1307. Edited by A. H. Thomas. Cambridge: Cambridge University Press, 1924.

Calendar of Letter-Books Preserved among the Archives of the Corporation of the City of London: Letter-Book K. Edited by R. R. Sharpe. London, 1911.

Calendar of the Liberate Rolls Preserved in the Public Record Office: Henry III. Vol. 3, A.D. 1245–1251. London: HMSO, 1937.

Calendar of the Patent Rolls Preserved in the Public Record Office: Edward III. Vol. 16, A.D. 1374–1377. London: HMSO, 1916.

Calendar of the Patent Rolls Preserved in the Public Record Office: Richard II. Vol. 1, A.D. 1377–1381. London: HMSO, 1895.

Calendar of the Patent Rolls Preserved in the Public Record Office: Richard II. Vol. 5, A.D. 1391–1396. London: HMSO, 1905.

Calendar of the Plea Rolls of the Exchequer of the Jews. Vol. 2, *Edward I, 1273–1275.* Edited by J. M. Rigg. Edinburgh: Ballantyne, Hanson and Co., 1910.

Calendar of Select Pleas and Memoranda of the City of London. Vol. 3. Edited by A. H. Thomas. Cambridge: Cambridge University Press, 1926.

Cartulary of St. Bartholomew's Hospital, Founded 1123. Edited by Nellie Kerling. London: Lund Humphries, 1973.

Cassiodorus. *Cassiodori Senatoris Institutiones.* Edited by R. A. B. Mynors. Oxford: Clarendon Press, 1937.

Cato. *Marcus Porcius Cato on Agriculture, Marcus Terentius Varro on Agriculture.* Translated by William Davis Hooper, revised by Harrison Boyd Ash. Loeb Classical Library. Cambridge, Mass.: Harvard University Press, 1954.

Chaucer, Geoffrey. *The Works of Geoffrey Chaucer.* Edited by F. N. Robinson. 2d ed. Boston: Houghton Mifflin, 1957.

Chaucer Life-Records. Edited by Martin M. Crow and Clair C. Olson from materials compiled by John M. Manly and Edith Rickert, with the assistance of Lilian J. Redstone and others. London: Oxford University Press, 1966.

The Chronicle of Melrose: A Complete and Full-Size Facsimile in Collotype. Introduction by Alan Orr Anderson and Marjorie Ogilvie Anderson, and an index by William Croft Dickinson. London: Percy Lund Humphries, 1936.

Chronicles of the Reigns of Stephen, Henry II, and Richard II. Vol 1, *Containing the First Four Books of the* Historia Rerum Anglicarum *of William of Newburgh.* Edited by Richard Howlett. Rolls Series 82. 1884. Reprint, Nendeln: Kraus, 1964.

Chronicon monasterii de Abingdon. Edited by Joseph Stevenson. Rolls Series vol. 2, pt. 2. London: Longman, 1858.

The Cutting Edge: Early History of the Surgeons of London. Edited by R. Theodore Beck. London: Lund Humphries, 1974.

Daniel, Henry. "A Critical Edition of the Middle English *Liber Uricrisiarum* in Wellcome MS 225." Edited by Joanne Jasin. Ph.D. diss., Tulane University, 1983.

Dante Alighieri. *Dante's Treatise "De Vulgari Eloquentia."* Translated by A. G. Ferrers Howell. London: Kegan Paul, 1890.

———. *De vulgari eloquentia.* Edited by Airstide Marigo. Florence: Felice Le Monnier, 1948.

The Dicts and Sayings of the Philosophers. Edited by Curt F. Bühler. Early English Text Society, o.s., 211. 1941. Reprint, London: Oxford University Press, 1961.

Early English Meals and Manners. Edited by Frederick J. Furnivall. Early English Text Society, o.s., 32. 1868. Reprint, London: N. Trubner, 1904.

Fleta. Vol. 2. Edited by H. G. Richardson and G. O. Sayles. Selden Society 72. London: B. Quaritch, 1955.

Gaddesden, John. *Rosa anglica practica a capite ad pedes.* Pavia, 1492.

Geohegan, D. "A Licence of Henry VI to Practise Alchemy." *Ambix* 6 (1957): 10–17.

Gilbertus Anglicus. *Compendium medicine.* Lyons: J. Saccon for V. de Portonariis, 1510.

Gower, John. *Latin Verses in the* Confessio Amantis: *An Annotated Translation.* Edited by Sian Echard and Claire Fanger. East Lansing, Mich. Colleagues Press, 1991.

Guy de Chauliac. *The Cyrurgie of Guy de Chauliac.* Edited by Margaret Ogden. Early English Text Society 265. London and New York: Oxford University Press, 1971.

———. *Guigonis de Caulhiaco (Guy de Chauliac): Inventarium sive Chirurgia Magna.* Vol. 1. Edited by Michael R. McVaugh. Leiden: E. J. Brill, 1997.

Hippocrates. *Hippocratic Writings.* Edited by G. E. R. Lloyd. New York: Penguin Books, 1978.

Hoccleve, Thomas. *The Regement of Princes A.D. 1411–12.* Edited by F. J. Furnivall. Early English Text Society, e.s. 72. London: K. Paul, Trench, Trubner, 1897.

Introduction to the Curia Regis Rolls, 1199–1230. Edited by C. T. Flower. Selden Society 62. London: B. Quaritch, 1944.

Isidore of Seville. *Etimologías: Edición Bilingüe.* Vol. 1. Edited and translated by José Oroz Reta and Manuel-A. Marcos Casquero. Madrid: Biblioteca de Autores Cristianos, 1982.

Isidore of Seville. "Isidore of Seville: The Medical Writings: An English Translation with an Introduction and Commentary." Edited by William D. Sharpe. *Transactions of the American Philosophical Society,* n.s., vol. 54, pt. 2. Philadelphia, 1964.

John of Mirfield. *Johannes de Mirfeld of St Bartholomew's, Smithfield: His Life and Works.* Edited by Percival Horton-Smith Hartley and Harold Richard Aldridge. Cambridge: Cambridge University Press, 1936.

———. *John of Mirfield (d. 1407), Surgery: A Translation of his* Breviarium Bartholomei, *Part IX.* Edited by James B. Colton. New York: Hafner, 1969.

A Latin Technical Phlebotomy and Its Middle English Translation. Edited by Linda E. Voigts and Michael R. McVaugh. *Transactions of the American Philosophical Society* 74, pt. 2. Philadelphia, 1984.

Leechdoms, Wortcunning and Starcraft of Early England. Vol. 2. Edited by Thomas Oswald Cockayne. 1865. Reprint, London: Holland Press, 1961.

Leet Jurisdiction in the City of Norwich during the xiiith and xivth Centuries. Edited by William Hudson. Selden Society 5. London: B. Quaritch, 1892.

Liber Niger Scaccarii. Vol. 2. Edited by Thomas Hearn. London, 1774.

The London Eyre of 1276. Edited by Martin Weinbaum. Leicester: London Records Society, 1976.

Lydgate, John. "John Lydgate's Dietary." Edited by Max Forster. *Anglia* 42 (1918): 176–91.

———. *The Minor Poems of John Lydgate.* Pt. 2, *Secular Poems.* Edited by Henry Noble MacCracken. Early English Text Society, o.s., 192. 1934. Reprint, London: Oxford University Press,1961.

Matthew Paris. *Gesta abbatum: Chronicles of Matthew Paris: Monastic Life in the Thirteenth Century.* Edited, translated and with an introduction by Richard Vaughn. New York: St. Martin's Press, 1984.

———. *Matthaei Parisiensis, Monachi Sancti Albani, Chronica Majora.* Vol. 4, A.D. *1240–1247.* Edited by Henry Richards Luard. Rolls Series 57. London: Longman, 1877.

Memorials of London and London Life. Edited by Henry T. Riley. London: Longman, 1868.

The Mirror of Justices. Edited by William Joseph Whittaker. Selden Society 7. London: B. Quaritch, 1895.

Monumenta Franciscana. Edited by J. S. Brewer. Rolls Series 1, pt. 4 1858. Reprint, Nendeln: Kraus, 1965.

Norton, Thomas. *Thomas Norton's Ordinal of Alchemy.* Edited by J. Reidy. Early English Text Society 272. London and New York: Oxford University Press, 1975.

Orderic Vitalis. *The Ecclesiastical History of Orderic Vitalis,* Vol. 2, *Books III and IV.* Edited and translated by Marjorie Chibnall. Oxford: Clarendon Press, 1969.

———. *The Ecclesiastical History of Orderic Vitalis.* Vol. 3, *Books V and VI.* Edited and trans. by Marjorie Chibnall. Oxford: Clarendon Press, 1972.

Patrologiae Cursus Completus: Series Latina. Vol. 89. Paris: J.-P. Migne, 1850.

The Peasants' Revolt of 1381. Edited by R. B. Dobson. London: Macmillan, 1970.

Petrarch, *Invectiva contra medicum: Testo latino e volgarizzamento di Ser Domenico Silvestri.* Edited by Pier Giorgio Ricci. Rome: Storia e Letteratura, 1950.

Pliny. *Natural History, with an English Translation in Ten Volumes.* Vol. 7. Edited by W. H. S. Jones. Loeb Classical Library. Cambridge, Mass.: Harvard University Press, 1966.

———. *Natural History, with an English Translation in Ten Volumes.* Vol. 8. Edited by W. H. S. Jones. Loeb Classical Library. Cambridge, Mass.: Harvard University Press, 1975.

Popular Medicine in Thirteenth-Century England: Introduction and Texts. Edited by Tony Hunt. Cambridge, England: D. S. Brewer, 1990.

Promptorium Parvulorum Sive Clericorum. Edited by Albertus Way. Camden Society, 1843.

Public Works in Mediaeval Law. Vol. 1. Edited by C. T. Flower. Selden Society 32. London: B. Quaritch, 1915.

Public Works in Mediaeval Law. Vol. 2. Edited by C. T. Flower. Selden Society 40. London: B. Quaritch, 1923.

Ralph of Coggeshall. *Radulphi de Coggeshall Chronicon Anglicanum.* Edited by Joseph Stevenson. Rolls Series 66. London: Longman, 1875.

Roger of Hovedene. *Chronica Magistri Rogeri de Houedene.* Edited by William Stubbs. Rolls Series 51, vol. 4. 1871. Reprint, Nendeln: Kraus, 1964.

The Roll of the Shropshire Eyre of 1256. Edited by Alan Harding. Selden Society 96. London, 1981.

Rolls of the Justices in Eyre being the Rolls of Pleas and Assizes for Gloucestershire, Warwickshire, and Staffordshire, 1221, 1222. Edited by Doris Mary Stenton. Selden Society 59. London: B. Quaritch, 1940.

Rolls of the Justices in Eyre being the Rolls of Pleas and Assizes for Yorkshire in 3 Henry III (1218–19). Edited by Doris Mary Stenton. Selden Society 56. London: B. Quaritch, 1937.

Rotuli parliamentorum. Vol. 4. London, n.d.

The Rule of St. Benedict: In Latin and English with Notes. Edited by Timothy Fry et al. Collegeville, Minn.: The Liturgical Press, 1981.

Secretum Secretorum: Nine English Versions. Edited by M. A. Manzalaoui. Early English Text Society 276. Oxford: Oxford University Press, 1977.

Select Cases in Chancery A.D. 1364 to 1471. Edited by William Paley Baildon. Selden Society 10. London: B. Quaritch, 1896.

Select Cases Concerning the Law Merchant A.D. 1270–1638. Vol. 1, *Local Courts.* Edited by Charles Gross. Selden Society 23. London: B. Quaritch, 1908.

Select Cases from the Coroners' Rolls A.D. 1265–1413. Edited by Charles Gross. Selden Society 9. London: B. Quaritch, 1896.

Select Cases in the Court of King's Bench under Edward I. Vol. 1. Edited by G. O. Sayles. Selden Society 55. London: B. Quaritch, 1936.

Select Cases in the Court of King's Bench under Edward I. Vol. 2. Edited by G. O. Sayles. Selden Society 57. London: B. Quaritch, 1938.

Select Cases in the Court of King's Bench under Edward I. Vol. 3. Edited by G. O. Sayles. Selden Society 58. London: B. Quaritch, 1939.

Select Cases in the Court of King's Bench under Edward III. Vol. 4. Edited by G. O. Sayles. Selden Society 82. London: B. Quaritch, 1965.

Select Cases in the Court of King's Bench under Richard II, Henry IV, and Henry V. Edited by G. O. Sayles. Selden Society 88. London: B. Quaritch, 1971.

Select Cases of Trespass from the King's Courts, 1307–1399. Vol. 1. Edited by Morris S. Arnold. Selden Society 100. London, 1985.

Select Cases of Trespass from the King's Courts, 1307–1399. Vol. 2. Edited by Morris S. Arnold. Selden Society 103. London, 1987.

Select Pleas of the Crown. Vol. 1, A.D. *1200–1225.* Edited by F. W. Maitland. Selden Society 1. London: B. Quaritch, 1888.

Seneca. *Seneca ad Lucilium Epistulae Morales.* Translated by Richard M. Gummere. Vol. 3. Loeb Classical Library. New York: Putnam's Sons, 1925.

Shetarot: Hebrew Deeds of English Jews before 1290. Edited by M. D. Davis. Publications of the Anglo-Jewish Historical Exhibition 2. London, 1888.

Sinonoma Bartholomei: A Glossary from a Fourteenth-Century Manuscript in the Library of Pembroke College, Oxford. Edited by J. L. G. Mowat. Oxford: Clarendon Press, 1882.

A Source Book in Medieval Science. Edited by Edward Grant. Cambridge, Mass.: Harvard University Press, 1974.

South, John Flint. *Memorials of the Craft of Surgery in England.* Edited by D'Arcy Power. London: Cassell and Co., 1886.

Theodoric of Lucca. *The Surgery of Theodoric.* Translated by Eldridge Campbell and James Colton. Vol. 2. New York: Appleton-Century-Crofts, 1960.

Thomas Walsingham. *Gesta Abbatum Monasterii Sancti Albani, a Thoma Walsingham.* Edited by Henry Thomas Riley. Vol. 1, A.D. *793–1290.* Rolls Series 28, vol. 1, pt. 4. London: Longman, 1867.

William of Malmesbury. *Willelmi Malmesbiriensis monachi de gestis pontificum anglorum.* Edited by N. E. S. A. Hamilton. Rolls Series 52. 1870. Reprint, Nendeln: Kraus, 1965.

———. *Willelmi Malmesbiriensis monachi de gestis regum anglorum libri quinque.* Edited by William Stubbs. Rolls Series 90, Vol. 1. London: HMSO, 1889.

Year Books of Edward II. Vol. 5, The Eyre of Kent 6&7 Edward II, A.D. *1313–1314.* Vol. 1. Edited by Frederic William Maitland, Leveson William Vernon Harcourt, and William Craddock Bolland. Selden Society 24. London: B. Quaritch, 1910.

Year Books of Edward II: The Eyre of London 14 Edward II, A.D. 1321. Vol. 1. Edited by Helen M. Cam. Selden Society 85. London: B. Quaritch, 1968.

Year Books of Edward II: The Eyre of London 14 Edward II, A.D. 1321. Vol. 2. Edited by Helen M. Cam. Selden Society 86. London: B. Quaritch, 1969.

Secondary Sources

Abelson, Paul. *The Seven Liberal Arts: A Study in Mediaeval Culture.* New York: Russell and Russell, 1906, reissued 1965.

Adams, J. N., and Marilyn Deegan. "Bald's *Leechbook* and the *Physica Plinii.*" *Anglo-Saxon England* 21 (1992): 87–114.

Adelard of Bath: An English Scientist and Arabist of the Early Twelfth Century. Edited by Charles Burnett. London: The Warburg Institute, 1987.

Agrimi, Jole, and Chiara Crisciani. "Medicina del corpo e medicina dell'anima: Note sul sapere del medico fino all'inizio del sec. XIII." *Episteme* 10 (1976): 5–102.

Albertus Magnus and the Sciences: Commemorative Essays. Edited by J. A. Weisheipl. Toronto: Pontifical Institute of Mediaeval Studies, 1980.

Alford, John A. "Medicine in the Middle Ages: The Theory of a Profession." *Centennial Review* 23 (1979): 377–96.

Allmand, C. T. "A Note on Denization in Fifteenth Century England." *Medievalia et Humanistica* 17 (1966): 127–28.

Alteras, Isaac. "Notes généalogiques sur les médecins juifs dans le sud de la France pendant les XIIIe et XIVe siècles." *Le moyen âge* 88 (1982): 29–47.

Amundsen, Darrel W. "History of Medical Ethics: Medieval Europe: Fourth to Sixteenth Century." In *The Encyclopedia of Bioethics*, edited by Warren T. Reich, 3;938–51. New York: The Free Press, 1978.

———. "Medieval Canon Law on Medical and Surgical Practice by the Clergy." *Bulletin of the History of Medicine* 52 (1978): 22–44.

Amundsen, Darrel W. and Gary B. Ferngren. "The Early Christian Tradition." In *Caring and Curing: Health and Medicine in the Western Religious Traditions*, edited by Ronald L. Numbers and Darrel W. Amundsen, 40–64. New York: Macmillan, 1986.

Anawati, G. "Medicine." In *The Cambridge History of Islam*, edited by P. M. Holt, Ann K. S. Lambton, and Bernard Lewis, 2;765–79. Cambridge: Cambridge University Press, 1970.

Anglo-Norman Dictionary. Edited by Louise W. Stone and William Rothwell. London: The Modern Humanities Research Association, 1985.

Arbesman, Ralph. "The Concept of 'Christus Medicus' in St. Augustine." *Traditio* 10 (1954): 1–28.

Auden, G. A. "The Gild of Barber Surgeons of the City of York." *Proceedings of the Royal Society of Medicine* 21, 2 (1928): 1400–1406.

Baader, Gerhard. "Medizin und Renaissancehumanismus." In *Istoriga dalla Madaschegna: Festschrift für Nikolaus Mani*, edited by Friedrun R. Hau, Gundolf Keil, and Charlotte Schubert, 115–39. Hannover: Horst Wellm Verlag, 1985.

———. "Die Tradition des Corpus Hippocraticum im europäischen Mittelalter." *Sudhoffs Archiv* Beiheft 27 (1989): 409–19.

Bailey, Mark. "Demographic Decline in Late Medieval England: Some Thoughts on Recent Research." *Economic History Review* 49 (1996): 1–19.

Baker, Robert L. "The English Customs Service, 1307–1343: A Study of Medieval Administration." *Transactions of the American Philosophical Society*, n.s., 51, pt. 6. Philadelphia, 1961.

Barlow, Frank. *The English Church, 1066–1154.* New York: Longman, 1979.

Barnes, Jonathan. "Galen on Logic and Therapy." In *Galen's Method of Healing: Proceedings of the 1982 Galen Symposium*, edited by Fridolf Kudlien and Richard J. Durling, 50–102. Leiden: E. J. Brill, 1991.

Barnet, Margaret C. "The Barber-Surgeons of York." *Medical History* 12 (1968): 19–30.

Beardwood, Alice. *Alien Merchants in England 1350 to 1377: Their Legal Status and Economic Position.* Cambridge, Mass.: Mediaeval Academy of America, 1931.

———. "Mercantile Antecedents of the English Naturalization Laws." *Medievalia et Humanistica* 16 (1964): 64–76.

Bell, Rudolph. *Holy Anorexia.* Chicago: University of Chicago Press, 1985.

Bennett, Judith M. "Medieval Women, Modern Women: Across the Great Divide." In *Culture and History, 1350–1600: Essays on English Communities, Identities and Writing*, edited by David Aers, 147–75. London: Harvester Wheatsheaf, 1992.

Benton, John F. "Trotula, Women's Problems, and the Professionalization of Medicine in the Middle Ages." *Bulletin of the History of Medicine* 59 (1985): 30–53.

Bethell, Denis. "The Making of a Twelfth-Century Relic Collection." *Studies in Church History* 8 (1972): 61–72.

———. "The Miracles of St. Ithamar." *Analecta Bollandiana* 89 (1971): 421–37.

Bloch, Herbert. *Monte Cassino in the Middle Ages*. Vol. 1. Cambridge, Mass.: Harvard University Press, 1986.

Bodden, Mary Catherine. "Evidence for Knowledge of Greek in Anglo-Saxon England." *Anglo-Saxon England* 17 (1988): 217–46.

Bono, James J. *The Word of God and the Languages of Man: Interpreting Nature in Early Modern Science and Medicine*. Vol. 1, *Ficino to Descartes*. Madison: University of Wisconsin Press, 1995.

Bonser, Wilfrid. *The Medical Background of Anglo-Saxon England: A Study in History, Psychology, and Folklore*. London: Wellcome Historical Medical Library, 1963.

Boswell, John. *Christianity, Social Tolerance, and Homosexuality: Gay People in Western Europe from the Beginning of the Christian Era to the Fourteenth Century*. Chicago: University of Chicago Press, 1980.

Boutcher, Warren. "Vernacular Humanism in the Sixteenth Century." In *The Cambridge Companion to Renaissance Humanism*, edited by Jill Kraye, 189–202. Cambridge: Cambridge University Press, 1996.

Bray, Jennifer R. "Concepts of Sainthood in Fourteenth-Century England." *Bulletin of the John Rylands University Library of Manchester* 66 (1983–84): 40–77.

Brody, Saul Nathaniel. *The Disease of the Soul: Leprosy in Medieval Literature*. Ithaca, N.Y.: Cornell University Press, 1974.

Brown, Peter. *The Cult of Saints: Its Rise and Function in Latin Christianity*. Chicago: University of Chicago Press, 1981.

Büchler, Alfred. "A Twelfth-Century Physician's Desk Book: The *Secreta Secretorum* of Petrus Alphonsi Quondam Moses Sephardi." *Journal of Jewish Studies* 37 (1986): 206–12.

Bullough, Vern L. "Duke Humphrey and His Medical Collections." *Renaissance News* 14 (1961): 87–91.

———. "The Mediaeval Medical School at Cambridge." *Mediaeval Studies* 24 (1962): 161–68.

———. "Medical Study at Mediaeval Oxford." *Speculum* 36 (1961): 600–612.

———. "Training of the Nonuniversity-Educated Medical Practitioners in the Later Middle Ages." *Journal of the History of Medicine* 14 (1959): 446–58.

Burnett, Charles S. F. "Some Comments on the Translating of Works from Arabic into Latin in the Mid-Twelfth Century." In *Orientalische Kultur und Europäisches Mittelalter*, edited by Albert Zimmermann, Berlin: Walter De Gruyter, 161–71. Miscellanea Mediaevalia 17. 1985.

Burrow, J. A. *Thomas Hoccleve*. Aldershot: Variorum, 1994.

Bylebyl, Jerome J. "The Medical Meaning of *Physica*." *Osiris*, 2d ser., 6 (1990): 16–41.

———. "Medicine, Philosophy, and Humanism in Renaissance Italy." In *Science and the Arts in the Renaissance*, edited by John W. Shirley and F. David Hoeniger, 27–49. Washington, D.C.: The Folger Shakespeare Library, 1985.

Bynum, Caroline Walker. *Holy Feast and Holy Fast: The Religious Significance of Food to Medieval Women*. Berkeley: University of California Press, 1987.

————. *The Resurrection of the Body in Western Christianity, 200–1336.* New York: Columbia University Press, 1995.

Cadden, Joan. *Meanings of Sex Difference in the Middle Ages: Medicine, Science, and Culture.* Cambridge: Cambridge University Press, 1993.

Cameron, M. L. *Anglo-Saxon Medicine.* Cambridge: Cambridge University Press, 1993.

————. "Bald's *Leechbook*: Its Sources and Their Use in Its Compilation." *Anglo-Saxon England* 12 (1983): 153–82.

————. "Bald's *Leechbook* and Cultural Interactions in Anglo-Saxon England." *Anglo-Saxon England* 19 (1990): 5–12.

————. "The Sources of Medical Knowledge in Anglo-Saxon England." *Anglo-Saxon England* 11 (1983): 135–55.

Carlin, Martha. "Medieval English Hospitals." In *The Hospital in History*, edited by Lindsay Granshaw and Roy Porter, 21–37. London: Routledge, 1989.

————. *Medieval Southwark.* London: The Hambledon Press, 1996.

Carroll, Clare. "Humanism and English Literature in the Fifteenth Century." In *The Cambridge Companion to Renaissance Humanism*, edited by Jill Kraye, 189–202, 246–68. Cambridge: Cambridge University Press, 1996.

Chazan, Robert. *Daggers of Faith: Thirteenth-Century Christian Missionizing and Jewish Response.* Berkeley: University of California Press, 1989.

————. *Medieval Jewry in Northern France: A Political and Social History.* Baltimore, Md.: The Johns Hopkins University Press, 1973.

Chibnall, Marjorie. "Pliny's *Natural History* and the Middle Ages." In *Empire and Aftermath: Silver Latin II*, edited by T. A. Dorey, 57–78. London: Routledge and Kegan Paul, 1975.

Cholmeley, H. P. *John of Gaddesden and the Rosa Medicinae.* Oxford: Clarendon Press, 1912.

Clark, Elaine. "Some Aspects of Social Security in Medieval England." *Journal of Family History* 7 (1982): 307–20.

Clarke, M. L. *Higher Education in the Ancient World.* London: Routledge and Kegan Paul, 1971.

Codices Latini Antiquiores: A Palaeographical Guide to Latin Manuscripts Prior to the Ninth Century. 2d ed. Edited by E. A. Lowe, revised by Virginia Brown. Oxford: Clarendon Press, 1972.

Cohen, Jeremy. *The Friars and the Jews: The Evolution of Medieval Anti-Judaism.* Ithaca, N.Y.: Cornell University Press, 1982.

Cohn-Sherbok, D. "Medieval Jewish Persecution in England: The Canterbury Pogroms in Perspective." *Southern History* 3 (1981): 23–37.

Companion Encyclopedia of the History of Medicine. Vol. 2. Edited by W. F. Bynum and Roy Porter. London: Routledge, 1993.

Cook, Harold J. *The Decline of the Old Medical Regime in Stuart London.* Ithaca, N.Y.: Cornell University Press, 1986.

————. *Trials of an Ordinary Doctor: Joannes Groenevelt in Seventeenth-Century London.* Baltimore, Md.: The Johns Hopkins University Press, 1994.

Corpus of British Medieval Library Catalogues: The Friars' Libraries. Edited by K. W. Humphreys. London: British Library, 1990.

Cosman, Madeleine Pelner. "Medieval Medical Malpractice: The Dicta and the Dockets." *Bulletin of the New York Academy of Medicine*, 2d ser., 49 (1973): 22–47.

Courtenay, William J. *Schools and Scholars in Fourteenth-Century England.* Princeton, N.J.: Princeton University Press, 1987.

Crisciani, Chiara. "History, Novelty, and Progress in Scholastic Medicine." *Osiris,* 2d ser., 6 (1990): 118–39.

D'Alverny, Marie-Thérèse. "Translations and Translators." In *Renaissance and Renewal in the Twelfth Century,* edited by Robert L. Benson and Giles Constable, with Carol D. Lanham, 421–62. Cambridge, Mass.: Harvard University Press, 1982.

D'Aronco, Maria Amalia. "The Botanical Lexicon of the Old English *Herbarium.*" *Anglo-Saxon England* 17 (1988): 15–33.

Dawtry, Anne F. "The *Modus Medendi* and the Benedictine Order in Anglo-Norman England." *Studies in Church History* 19 (1982): 25–38.

De La Mare, A. C. "Manuscripts Given to the University of Oxford by Humfrey, Duke of Gloucester." *Bodleian Library Record* 13, 1 (1988): 30–51; 13, 2 (1989): 112–21.

Demaitre, Luke E. *Doctor Bernard de Gordon: Professor and Practitioner.* Toronto: Pontifical Institute of Mediaeval Studies, 1980.

———. "Scholasticism in Compendia of Practical Medicine, 1250–1450." *Manuscripta* 20 (1976): 81–95.

Dictionary of Medieval Latin from British Sources. Prepared by R. E. Latham. London: Oxford University Press for the British Academy, 1975.

Dictionary of Scientific Biography. Charles Coulston Gillispie, editor-in-chief. New York: Charles Scribner's Sons, 1970–90.

Dobson, Jessie, and R. Milnes Walker. *Barbers and Barber-Surgeons of London: A History of the Barbers' and Barber-Surgeons' Companies.* Oxford: Blackwell Scientific Publications, 1979.

Dobson, R. B. "Admissions to the Freedom of the City of York in the Later Middle Ages." *Economic History Review* 26 (1973): 1–21.

———. "The Decline and Expulsion of the Medieval Jews of York." *Jewish Historical Studies: Transactions of the Jewish Historical Society of England* 26 (1974–78): 34–52.

———. "The Jews of Medieval Cambridge." *Jewish Historical Studies: Transactions of the Jewish Historical Society of England* 32 (1990–92): 1–24.

Duncan, Edgar H. "The Literature of Alchemy and Chaucer's Canon's Yeoman's Tale: Framework, Theme, and Characters." *Speculum* 43 (1968): 633–56.

Eamon, William. *Science and the Secrets of Nature: Books of Secrets in Medieval and Early Modern Culture.* Princeton, N.J.: Princeton University Press, 1994.

Eamon, William, and Gundolf Keil. " 'Plebs amat empirica': Nicholas of Poland and His Critique of the Medieval Medical Establishment." *Sudhoffs Archiv* 71 (1987): 180–96.

Edelstein, Ludwig. *Ancient Medicine: Selected Papers of Ludwig Edelstein.* Edited by Owsei Temkin and C. Lilian Temkin. Baltimore, Md.: The Johns Hopkins University Press, 1967.

Ellis, Roger. "The English Lands and Revenues of Master Pancio da Controne." *Rivista di storia delle scienze mediche e naturali* 43 (1952): 266–74.

Emden, A. B. *A Biographical Register of the University of Cambridge to 1500.* Cambridge: Cambridge University Press, 1963.

———. *A Biographical Register of the University of Oxford to 1500.* 3 vols. Oxford: Clarendon Press, 1957–59.

Emery, Richard W. "Jewish Physicians in Medieval Perpignan." *Michael: On the History of the Jews in the Diaspora* 12 (1991): 113–34.

Fichtner, Gerhard. "Christus als Arzt. Ursprünge und Wirkungen eines Motivs." *Frühmittelalterliche Studien* 16 (1982): 1–18.

Finucane, Ronald C. *Miracles and Pilgrims: Popular Beliefs in Medieval England.* Totowa, N.J.: Rowman and Littlefield, 1977.

———. "The Use and Abuse of Medieval Miracles." *History* 60 (1975): 1–10.

Forbes, Thomas R. "A Jury of Matrons." *Medical History* 32 (1988): 23–33.

French, Roger. *Ancient Natural History: Histories of Nature.* London: Routledge, 1994.

Gabrieli, F. "The Transmission of Learning." In *The Cambridge History of Islam,* edited by P. M. Holt, Ann K. S. Lambton, and Bernard Lewis, 2:851–68. Cambridge: Cambridge University Press, 1970.

Gask, George. "The Medical Services of Henry the Fifth's Campaign of the Somme in 1415." In *Essays in the History of Medicine,* 94–102. London: Butterworth, 1950.

Geary, Patrick J. *Living with the Dead in the Middle Ages.* Ithaca, N.Y.: Cornell University Press, 1994.

Getz, Faye Marie. "Black Death and the Silver Lining: Meaning, Continuity, and Revolutionary Change in Histories of Medieval Plague." *Journal of the History of Biology* 24 (1991): 265–89.

———. "Charity, Translation, and the Language of Medical Learning in Medieval England." *Bulletin of the History of Medicine* 64 (1990): 1–17.

———. "The Faculty of Medicine before 1500." In *The History of the University of Oxford,* vol. 2, *Late Medieval Oxford,* edited by Jeremy Catto and Ralph Evans, 373–405. Oxford: Clarendon Press, 1992.

———. "John Mirfield and the *Breviarium Bartholomei*: The Medical Writings of a Clerk at St Bartholomew's Hospital in the Later Fourteenth Century." *Society for the Social History of Medicine Bulletin* 37 (1985): 24–26.

———. "Medical Education in Later Medieval England." In *The History of Medical Education in Britain,* edited by Vivian Nutton and Roy Porter, 76–93. Amsterdam: Rodopi, 1995.

———. "Medical Practitioners in Medieval England." *Social History of Medicine* 3 (1990): 245–83.

———. "The *Method of Healing* in Middle English." In *Galen's Method of Healing: Proceedings of the 1982 Galen Symposium,* edited by Fridolf Kudlien and Richard J. Durling, 147–56. Leiden: E. J. Brill, 1991.

———. "To Prolong Life and Promote Health: Baconian Alchemy and Pharmacy in the English Learned Tradition." In *Health, Disease and Healing in Medieval Culture,* edited by Sheila Campbell, Bert Hall, and David Klausner, 141–51. New York: St. Martin's Press, 1992.

Getz, Faye Marie, ed. *Healing and Society in Medieval England: A Middle English Translation of the Pharmaceutical Writings of Gilbertus Anglicus.* Madison: University of Wisconsin Press, 1991.

Gordon, Eleanora. "Accidents among Medieval Children as Seen from the Miracles of Six English Saints and Martyrs." *Medical History* 35 (1991): 145–63.

———. "Child Health in the Middle Ages as Seen in the Miracles of Five English Saints, A.D. 1150–1220." *Bulletin of the History of Medicine* 60 (1986): 502–22.

Gottfried, Robert S. *Doctors and Medicine in Medieval England, 1340–1530.* Princeton, N.J.: Princeton University Press, 1986.

Gracia, Diego. "The Structure of Medical Knowledge in Aristotle's Philosophy." *Sudhoffs Archiv* 62 (1978): 1–36.

Green, Monica. "Obstetrical and Gynecological Texts in Middle English." *Studies in the Age of Chaucer* 14 (1992): 53–88.

———. "Women's Medical Practice and Health Care in Medieval Europe." *Signs* 14 (1989): 434–73.

Hammond, E. A. "Incomes of Medieval English Doctors." *Journal of the History of Medicine* 15 (1960): 154–69.

———. "Physicians in Medieval English Religious Houses." *Bulletin of the History of Medicine* 32 (1958): 105–20.

———. "The Westminster Abbey Infirmarers' Rolls as a Source of Medical History." *Bulletin of the History of Medicine* 39 (1965): 261–76.

Hanawalt, Barbara A. *Growing up in Medieval London: The Experience of Childhood in History.* New York: Oxford University Press, 1993.

Handerson, Henry E. *Gilbertus Anglicus: Medicine of the Thirteenth Century.* Cleveland, Ohio: Cleveland Medical Library Association, 1918.

Hanna III, Ralph. "Henry Daniel's *Liber Uricrisiarum* (Excerpt)." In *Popular and Practical Science of Medieval England*, edited by Lister M. Matheson, 185–218. East Lansing, Mich.: Colleagues Press, 1994.

Harvey, Barbara. *Living and Dying in England, 1100–1540: The Monastic Experience.* Oxford: Clarendon Press, 1993.

Hatcher, John. *Plague, Population and the English Economy, 1348–1530.* London: Macmillan, 1977.

Health, Medicine, and Mortality in the Sixteenth Century. Edited by Charles Webster. Cambridge: Cambridge University Press, 1979.

Helmholz, R. H. "Infanticide in the Province of Canterbury during the Fifteenth Century." *History of Childhood Quarterly* 2 (1974–75): 379–90.

Heresy and Literacy, 1000–1530. Edited by Peter Biller and Anne Hudson. Cambridge: Cambridge University Press, 1994.

Hillaby, Joe. "London: The 13th-Century Jewry Revisited." *Jewish Historical Studies: Transactions of the Jewish Historical Society of England* 32 (1990–92): 89–158.

———. "A Magnate among the Marchers: Hamo of Hereford, His Family and Clients, 1218–1253." *Jewish Historical Studies: Transactions of the Jewish Historical Society of England* 31 (1988–90): 23–82.

Hirsch, S. A. "Roger Bacon and Philology." In *Roger Bacon Essays*, edited by A. G. Little, 101–51. Oxford: Clarendon Press, 1914.

Hollister, C. Warren. "Courtly Culture and Courtly Style in the Anglo-Norman World." *Albion* 20 (1988): 1–17.

Hudson, Anne. *The Premature Reformation: Wycliffite Texts and Lollard History.* Oxford: Clarendon Press, 1988.

Hunnisett, R. F. *The Medieval Coroner.* Cambridge: Cambridge University Press, 1961.

Hunt, R. W. "The Disputation of Peter of Cornwall against Symon the Jew." In *Studies in Medieval History Presented to Frederick Maurice Powicke*, edited by R. W. Hunt, W. A. Pantin, and R. W. Southern, 143–56. Oxford: Clarendon Press, 1948.

———. *The Schools and the Cloister: The Life and Writings of Alexander Nequam (1157–1217)*. Edited and revised by Margaret Gibson. Oxford: Clarendon Press, 1984.

Jacobs, Joseph. "Une lettre française d'un juif anglais au XIIIe siècle." *Revue des études juives* 18 (1889): 256–61.

Jacquart, Danielle. *Dictionnaire biographique des médecins en France au moyen âge: Supplément.* Geneva: Librairie Droz, 1979.

———. "The Introduction of Arabic Medicine into the West: The Question of Etiology." In *Health, Disease and Healing in Medieval Culture*, edited by Sheila Campbell, Bert Hall, and David Klausner, 186–95. New York: St. Martin's Press, 1992.

———. *Le milieu médical en France du XIIe au XVe siècle, en annexe 2e supplément au Dictionnaire d'Ernest Wickersheimer.* Geneva: Librairie Droz, 1981.

James, Montague Rhodes. *A Descriptive Catalogue of the Manuscripts in the Library of Peterhouse*. Cambridge: Cambridge University Press, 1899.

———. "Greek Manuscripts in England before the Renaissance." *The Library*, n.s., 7 (1927): 337–53.

Jasin, Joanne. "The Transmission of Learned Medical Literature in the Middle English *Liber Uricrisiarum*." *Medical History* 37 (1993): 313–29.

Jenks, Stuart. "Medizinische Fachkräfte in England zur Zeit Heinrichs VI (1428/29–1460/61)." *Sudhoffs Archiv* 69 (1985): 214–27.

Jones, Peter Murray. "Four Middle English Translations of John of Arderne." In *Latin and Vernacular: Studies in Late Medieval Manuscripts*, edited by Alastair Minnis, 61–89. Wolfeboro, N.H.: D. S. Brewer, 1989.

———. "John of Arderne and the Mediterranean Tradition of Scholastic Surgery." In *Practical Medicine from Salerno to the Black Death*, edited by Luis García-Ballester, Roger French, Jon Arrizabalaga, and Andrew Cunningham, 289–321. Cambridge: Cambridge University Press, 1994.

———. " 'Sicut hic depingitur . . .': John of Arderne and English Medical Illustration in the 14th and 15th Centuries." In *Die Kunst und das Studium der Natur vom 14. zum 16. Jahrhundert*, edited by Wolfram Prinz and Andreas Beyer, 103–26, 379–92. Weinheim: VCH, 1987.

Jordan, William Chester. *The Great Famine: Northern Europe in the Early Fourteenth Century.* Princeton, N.J.: Princeton University Press, 1996.

Kealey, Edward J. "England's Earliest Women Doctors." *Journal of the History of Medicine* 40 (1985): 473–77.

———. *Medieval Medicus: A Social History of Anglo-Norman Medicine.* Baltimore, Md.: The Johns Hopkins University Press, 1981.

Kellaway, William. "The Coroner in Medieval London." In *Studies in London History Presented to Philip Edmund Jones*, edited by A. E. J. Hollaender and William Kellaway, 75–91. London: Hodder and Stoughton, 1969.

Kellum, Barbara A. "Infanticide in England in the Later Middle Ages." *History of Childhood Quarterly* 1 (1973–74): 367–88.

Ker, N. R. *Catalogue of Manuscripts Containing Anglo-Saxon.* Oxford: Clarendon Press, 1957.

Kerling, Nellie. *Commercial Relations of Holland and Zeeland with England from the Late 13th Century to the Close of the Middle Ages.* Leiden: E. J. Brill, 1954.

Kershaw, Ian. "The Great Famine and Agrarian Crisis in England, 1315–1322." *Past and Present* no. 59 (1973): 3–50.

Kibre, Pearl. "Arts and Medicine in the Universities of the Later Middle Ages." In *The Universities in the Late Middle Ages*, edited by Jozef IJsewijn and Jacques Paquet, 213–77. Louvain: Leuven University Press, 1978.

———. "The Faculty of Medicine at Paris, Charlatanism and Unlicensed Medical Practice in the Later Middle Ages." *Bulletin of the History of Medicine* 27 (1953): 1–20.

———. *Hippocrates Latinus: Repertorium of Hippocratic Writings in the Latin Middle Ages*. Rev. ed. New York: Fordham University Press, 1985.

———. "The Intellectual Interests Reflected in Libraries of the Fourteenth and Fifteenth Centuries." In *Studies in Medieval Science: Alchemy, Astrology, Mathematics and Medicine*, 257–97. London: The Hambledon Press, 1984.

———. "Lewis of Caerleon, Doctor of Medicine, Astronomer, and Mathematician (d. 1494?)." *Isis* 43 (1952): 100–108.

Kristeller, Paul Oskar. "The School of Salerno: Its Development and Its Contribution to the History of Learning." *Bulletin of the History of Medicine* 17 (1945): 138–94.

Kudlien, Fridolf. "Medicine as a 'Liberal Art' and the Question of the Physician's Income." *Journal of the History of Medicine* 31 (1976): 448–59.

Kühnert, Friedmar. *Allgemeinbildung und Fachbildung in der Antike*. Berlin: Akademie-Verlag, 1961.

Lang, S. J. "John Bradmore and His Book *Philomena*." *Social History of Medicine* 5 (1992): 121–30.

Langmuir, Gavin I. "The Knight's Tale and Young Hugh of Lincoln." *Speculum* 47 (1972): 459–82.

———. "Thomas of Monmouth: Detector of Ritual Murder." *Speculum* 59 (1984): 820–46.

Larusso, Dominic A. "Rhetoric in the Italian Renaissance." In *Renaissance Eloquence: Studies in the Theory and Practice of Renaissance Rhetoric*, 37–55. Berkeley: University of California Press, 1983.

Lawton, David. "Dullness and the Fifteenth Century." *English Literary History* 54 (1987): 761–99.

Leader, Damian Riehl. *A History of the University of Cambridge*. Vol. 1, *The University to 1546*. Cambridge: Cambridge University Press, 1988.

Levine, Joseph M. *Humanism and History: Origins of Modern English Historiography*. Ithaca, N.Y.: Cornell University Press, 1987.

Lévi-Strauss, Claude. "The Sorcerer and His Magic." In *Structural Anthropology*, translated by Claire Jacobson and Brooke Grundfest Schoepf, 167–85. New York: Basic Books, 1963.

Liebeschütz, Hans. *Medieval Humanism in the Life and Writings of John of Salisbury*. London: The Warburg Institute, 1950.

Lipman, V. D. *The Jews of Medieval Norwich*. London: Jewish Historical Society of England, 1967.

Lloyd, G. E. R. *Magic, Reason and Experience: Studies in the Origin and Development of Greek Science*. Cambridge: Cambridge University Press, 1979.

———. *Science, Folklore and Ideology*. Cambridge: Cambridge University Press, 1983.

Lloyd, T. H. *Alien Merchants in England in the High Middle Ages*. New York: St. Martin's Press, 1982.

Lonie, Iain M. "Literacy and the Development of Hippocratic Medicine." In *Formes de pensée dans la Collection Hippocratique,* edited by F. Lasserre and P. Mudry, 145–61. Geneva: Librairie Droz, 1983.

Loschky, David, and Ben D. Childers. "Early English Mortality." *Journal of Interdisciplinary History* 24 (1993): 85–97.

Lyon, Bryce. *A Constitutional and Legal History of Medieval England.* New York: Harper and Row, 1960.

Lytle, Guy Fitch. "The Social Origins of Oxford Students in the Late Middle Ages: New College, c. 1380–1510." In *The Universities in the Late Middle Ages,* edited by Jozef IJsewijn and Jacques Paquet, 426–54. Louvain: Leuven University Press, 1978.

MacDonald, Michael, and Terence R. Murphy. *Sleepless Souls: Suicide in Early Modern England.* Oxford: Clarendon Press, 1990.

McGovern, Jr., William M. "The Enforcement of Informal Contracts in the Later Middle Ages." *California Law Review* 59 (1971): 1145–93.

McLaughlin, T. P. "The Teaching of the Canonists on Usury (XII, XIII and XIV Centuries)." *Mediaeval Studies* 1 (1939): 81–147.

McVaugh, Michael R. "An Early Discussion of Medicinal Degrees at Montpellier by Henry of Winchester." *Bulletin of the History of Medicine* 49 (1975): 57–71.

———. *Medicine before the Plague: Practitioners and Their Patients in the Crown of Aragon, 1285–1345.* Cambridge: Cambridge University Press, 1993.

———. "Quantified Medical Theory and Practice at Fourteenth-Century Montpellier." *Bulletin of the History of Medicine* 43 (1969): 397–413.

Maddison, Francis, Margaret Pelling, and Charles Webster. *Essays on the Life and Work of Thomas Linacre.* Oxford: Clarendon Press, 1977.

Marrou, H. I. *History of Education in Antiquity.* Translated by George Lamb. New York: Sheed and Ward, 1956.

Matthews, Leslie G. *The Royal Apothecaries.* London: Wellcome Historical Medical Library, 1967.

Meaney, Audrey. "King Alfred and His Secretariat." *Parergon* 11 (1975): 16–23.

———. "Variant Versions of Old English Medical Remedies and the Compilation of Bald's *Leechbook.*" *Anglo-Saxon England* 13 (1984): 235–68.

———. "Women, Witchcraft and Magic in Anglo-Saxon England." In *Superstition and Popular Medicine in Anglo-Saxon England,* edited by D. G. Scragg, 9–40. Manchester: Centre for Anglo-Saxon Studies, 1989.

Medieval Libraries of Great Britain; a List of Surviving Books. 2d ed. Edited by N. R. Ker. London: Royal Historical Society, 1964.

Medieval Libraries of Great Britain, a List of Surviving Books, edited by N. R. Ker, Supplement to the Second Edition. Edited by Andrew G. Watson. London: Royal Historical Society, 1987.

Metlitzki, Dorothee. *The Matter of Araby in Medieval England.* New Haven, Conn.: Yale University Press, 1977.

Middle English Dictionary. Ann Arbor: University of Michigan Press, 1956– .

Miller, Gordon L. "Literacy and the Hippocratic Art: Reading, Writing, and Epistemology in Ancient Greek Medicine." *Journal of the History of Medicine* 45 (1990): 11–40.

Milsom, S. F. C. "Reason in the Development of the Common Law." *Law Quarterly Review* 81 (Oct. 1965): 496–517.

Mitchell, Rosamond J. *John Free: From Bristol to Rome in the Fifteenth Century.* London: Longman, 1955.

Mundill, Robin. "Anglo-Jewry under Edward I: Credit Agents and their Clients." *Jewish Historical Studies: Transactions of the Jewish Historical Society of England* 31 (1988–90): 1–21.

———. "The Jewish Entries from the Patent Rolls, 1272–1292." *Jewish Historical Studies: Transactions of the Jewish Historical Society of England* 32 (1990–92): 25–88.

Munro, John H. "Bullionism and the Bill of Exchange in England, 1272–1663: A Study in Monetary Management and Popular Prejudice." In *The Dawn of Modern Banking,* 169–239. New Haven, Conn.: Yale University Press, 1979.

Murphy, James J. *Medieval Rhetoric: A Select Bibliography.* Toronto: University of Toronto Press, 1989.

Murray, Jacqueline. "On the Origins and Role of 'Wise Women' in Causes for Annulment on the Grounds of Male Impotence." *Journal of Medieval History* 16 (1990): 235–49.

Mustain, James K. "A Rural Medical Practitioner in Fifteenth-Century England." *Bulletin of the History of Medicine* 46 (1972): 469–76.

Mynors, R. A. B. *Catalogue of the Manuscripts of Balliol College Oxford.* Oxford: Clarendon Press, 1963.

Nauert, Jr., Charles G. *Humanism and the Culture of Renaissance Europe.* Cambridge: Cambridge University Press, 1995.

Neibyl, Peter H. "Sennert, Van Helmont, and Medical Ontology." *Bulletin of the History of Medicine* 45 (1971): 115–37.

North, J. D. "Astronomy and Mathematics." In *The History of the University of Oxford,* vol. 2, *Late Medieval Oxford,* edited by Jeremy Catto and Ralph Evans, 102–74. Oxford: Clarendon Press, 1992.

———. *Chaucer's Universe.* Oxford: Clarendon Press, 1988.

———. "Natural Philosophy in Late Medieval Oxford." In *The History of the University of Oxford,* vol. 2, *Late Medieval Oxford,* edited by Jeremy Catto and Ralph Evans, 65–102. Oxford: Clarendon Press, 1992.

Ogilvy, J. D. A. *Books Known to Anglo-Saxon Writers from Aldhelm to Alcuin (670–804).* Cambridge, Mass.: Mediaeval Academy of America, 1936.

Olsan, Lea T. "Latin Charms in British Library, MS Royal 12.B.XXV," *Manuscripta* 33 (1989): 119–28.

———. "Latin Charms of Medieval England: Verbal Healing in a Christian Oral Tradition." *Oral Tradition* 7 (1992): 116–42.

Orme, Nicholas. *Education and Society in Medieval and Renaissance England.* London: The Hambledon Press, 1989.

———. *English Schools in the Middle Ages.* London: Methuen, 1973.

Orme, Nicholas, and Margaret Webster. *The English Hospital, 1070–1570.* New Haven, Conn.: Yale University Press, 1995.

Paravicini Bagliani, Agostino. *Medicina e scienze della natura alla corte dei papi nel duecento.* Spoleto: Centro Italiano di Studi Sull'Alto Medioevo, 1991.

Park, Katharine. *Doctors and Medicine in Early Renaissance Florence.* Princeton, N.J.: Princeton University Press, 1985.

————. "The Life of the Corpse: Division and Dissection in Late Medieval Europe." *Journal of the History of Medicine* 50 (1995): 111–32.

Parkes, Malcolm B. "The Influence of the Concepts of *Ordinatio* and *Compilatio* on the Development of the Book." In *Medieval Learning and Literature: Essays Presented to Richard William Hunt,* edited by J. J. G. Alexander and M. T. Gibson, 115–41. Oxford: Clarendon Press, 1976.

————. "The Palaeography of the Parker Manuscript of the Chronicle, Laws and Sedulius, and Historiography at Winchester in the Late Ninth and Tenth Centuries." *Anglo-Saxon England* 5 (1976): 149–71.

Pearsall, Derek. "Hoccleve's *Regement of Princes*: The Poetics of Royal Self-Representation." *Speculum* 69 (1994): 386–410.

Pelling, Margaret. "Medical Practice in Early Modern England: Trade or Profession?" In *The Professions in Early Modern England,* edited by W. Prest, 90–128. London: Croom Helm, 1987.

————. "Occupational Diversity: Barbersurgeons and the Trades of Norwich, 1550–1640." *Bulletin of the History of Medicine* 56 (1982): 484–511.

Pelling, Margaret, and Charles Webster. "Medical Practitioners." In *Health, Medicine, and Mortality in the Sixteenth Century,* edited by Charles Webster, 165–235. Cambridge: Cambridge University Press, 1979.

Pereira, Michela. "Un tesoro inestimabile: Elixir e 'Prolongatio Vitae' nell'alchimia de '300." *Micrologus: I discorsi dei corpi* 1 (1993): 161–87.

Post, Gaines, Kimon Giocarinis, and Richard Kay. "The Medieval Heritage of a Humanistic Ideal: '*Scientia Donum Dei Est, unde Vendi Non Potest*'." *Traditio* 11 (1955): 195–234.

Pouchelle, Marie-Christiane. *The Body and Surgery in the Middle Ages.* Translated by Rosemary Morris. New Brunswick, N.J.: Rutgers University Press, 1990.

Power, Eileen. *Medieval English Nunneries, c. 1275–1535.* Cambridge: Cambridge University Press, 1922.

Prestwich, Michael. "Italian Merchants in Late Thirteenth and Early Fourteenth Century England." In *The Dawn of Modern Banking,* 77–104. New Haven, Conn.: Yale University Press, 1979.

Profession, Vocation, and Culture in Later Medieval England: Essays Dedicated to the Memory of A. R. Myers. Edited by Cecil Clough. Liverpool: Liverpool University Press, 1982.

Pseudo-Aristotle, The Secret of Secrets. Edited by W. F. Ryan and Charles B. Schmitt. London: The Warburg Institute, 1982.

Rather, L. J. " 'The Six Things Non-Natural': A Note on the Origins and Fate of a Doctrine and a Phrase." *Clio Medica* 3 (1968): 337–47.

Rawcliffe, Carole. "The Hospitals of Later Medieval London." *Medical History* 28 (1984): 1–21.

————. *Medicine and Society in Later Medieval England.* Stroud: Alan Sutton, 1995.

————. "The Profits of Practice: The Wealth and Status of Medical Men in Later Medieval England." *Social History of Medicine* 1 (1988): 61–78.

Reynolds, L. D., and N. G. Wilson. *Scribes and Scholars: A Guide to the Transmission of Greek and Latin Literature.* 2d ed. Oxford: Clarendon Press, 1974.

Richards, Peter. *The Medieval Leper and His Northern Heirs.* Cambridge, England: D. S. Brewer, 1977.

Richardson, H. G. *The English Jewry under Angevin Kings.* London: Methuen, 1960.

Robbins, Rossell Hope. "John Crophill's Ale-Pots." *Review of English Studies*, n.s., 20, no. 78 (1969): 182–89.

———. "Medical Manuscripts in Middle English." *Speculum* 45 (1970): 393–415.

Rokéah, Zefira Entin. "Money and the Hangman in Late-13th-Century England: Jews, Christians and Coinage Offences Alleged and Real (Part I)." *Jewish Historical Studies: Transactions of the Jewish Historical Society of England* 31 (1988–90): 83–109.

———. "Unnatural Child Death among Christians and Jews in Medieval England." *Journal of Psychohistory* 18 (1990–1991): 181–226.

Roth, Cecil. "Elijah of London: The Most Illustrious English Jew of the Middle Ages." *Transactions of the Jewish Historical Society of England* 15 (1939–45): 29–62.

———. *A History of the Jews in England*. 3d ed. Oxford: Clarendon Press, 1964.

———. "Jewish Physicians in Medieval England." *Medical Leaves* 5 (1943): 42–45.

———. *The Jews of Medieval Oxford*. Oxford Historical Society, n.s., 9. Oxford: Clarendon Press, 1951.

———. "The Middle Period of Anglo-Jewish History (1290–1655) Reconsidered." *Jewish Historical Society of England Transactions* 19 (1955–59): 1–3.

———. "The Qualification of Jewish Physicians in the Middle Ages." *Speculum* 28 (1953): 834–43.

Rothwell, William. "The Role of French in Thirteenth-Century England." *Bulletin of the John Rylands University Library* 58 (1975–76): 445–66.

Rubin, Miri. *Charity and Community in Medieval Cambridge*. Cambridge: Cambridge University Press, 1987.

———. "Development and Change in English Hospitals, 1100–1500." In *The Hospital in History*, edited by Lindsay Granshaw and Roy Porter, 41–59. London: Routledge, 1989.

Rubin, Stanley. *Medieval English Medicine*. New York: Barnes and Noble, 1974.

Scanlon, Larry. "The King's Two Voices: Narrative and Power in Hoccleve's *Regement of Princes*." In *Literary Practice and Social Change in Britain, 1380–1530*, edited by Lee Patterson, 216–47. Berkeley: University of California Press, 1990.

———. *Narrative, Authority, and Power: The Medieval Exemplum and the Chaucerian Tradition*. Cambridge: Cambridge University Press, 1994.

Schmitt, Jean-Claude. "Le suicide au moyen âge." *Annales E. S. C.* 31 (1976): 3–28.

Science in the Middle Ages. Edited by David C. Lindberg. Chicago: University of Chicago Press, 1978.

Scully, Terence. "The Sickdish in Early French Recipe Collections." In *Health, Disease and Healing in Medieval Culture*, edited by Sheila Campbell, Bert Hall, and David Klausner, 132–40. New York: St. Martin's Press, 1992.

Seymour, M. C., et al. *Bartholomaeus Anglicus and His Encyclopedia*. Aldershot: Variorum, 1992.

Sezgin, Fuat. "Hunain b. Ishaq." In *Geschichte des arabischen Schrifttums*, 3:247–56. Leiden: E. J. Brill, 1970.

Shahar, Shulamith. "The Old Body in Medieval Culture." In *Framing Medieval Bodies*, edited by Sarah Kay and Miri Rubin, 160–86. Manchester: Manchester University Press, 1994.

———. "Who Were Old in the Middle Ages." *Social History of Medicine* 6 (1993): 313–41.

Shatzmiller, Joseph. *Jews, Medicine, and Medieval Society.* Berkeley: University of California Press, 1994.

Siraisi, Nancy G. *Avicenna in Renaissance Italy.* Princeton, N.J.: Princeton University Press, 1987.

———. *Medieval and Early Renaissance Medicine: An Introduction to Knowledge and Practice.* Chicago: University of Chicago Press, 1990.

———. *Taddeo Alderotti and His Pupils: Two Generations of Italian Medical Learning.* Princeton, N.J.: Princeton University Press, 1981.

Southern, R. W. *Robert Grosseteste: The Growth of an English Mind in Medieval Europe.* Oxford: Clarendon Press, 1986.

———. *Scholastic Humanism and the Unification of Europe.* Vol. 1, *Foundations.* Oxford: Blackwell Publishers, 1995.

Streit, Kevin T. "The Expansion of the English Jewish Community in the Reign of King Stephen." *Albion* 25 (1993): 177–92.

Swanson, Heather. "The Illusion of Economic Structure: Craft Guilds in Late Medieval English Towns." *Past and Present* no. 121 (1988): 29–48.

Sylla, Edith. "Medieval Quantifications of Qualities: The 'Merton School.' " *Archive for History of Exact Sciences* 8 (1971): 9–29.

Talbot, C. H. *Medicine in Medieval England.* London: Oldbourne, 1967.

———. "Simon Bredon (c. 1300–1372), Physician, Mathematician and Astronomer." *British Journal for the History of Science* 1 (1962–63): 19–30.

Talbot, C. H., and E. A. Hammond. *The Medical Practitioners in Medieval England: A Biographical Register.* London: Wellcome Historical Medical Library, 1965.

Temkin, Owsei. *Galenism: Rise and Decline of a Medical Philosophy.* Ithaca, N.Y.: Cornell University Press, 1973.

———. *Hippocrates in a World of Pagans and Christians.* Baltimore, Md.: The Johns Hopkins University Press, 1991.

Thorndike, Lynn, and Pearl Kibre. *A Catalogue of Incipits of Mediaeval Scientific Writings in Latin.* London: Mediaeval Academy of America, 1963.

Thrupp, Sylvia L. "Aliens in and around London in the Fifteenth Century." In *Studies in London History Presented to Philip Edmund Jones,* edited by A. E. J. Hollaender and William Kellaway, 251–72. London: Hodder and Stoughton, 1969.

———. *The Merchant Class of Medieval London, 1300–1500.* Chicago: University of Chicago Press, 1948.

———. "A Survey of the Alien Population of England in 1440." *Speculum* 32 (1958): 262–73.

Tolan, John. *Petrus Alfonsi and His Medieval Readers.* Gainesville: University Press of Florida, 1993.

Trease, G. E. "The Spicers and Apothecaries of the Royal Household in the Reigns of Henry III, Edward I and Edward II." *Nottingham Mediaeval Studies* 3 (1959): 19–52.

Trease, G. E., and J. H. Hodson. "The Inventory of John Hexham, A Fifteenth-Century Apothecary." *Medical History* 9 (1965): 76–81.

Ullmann, Manfred. *Islamic Medicine.* Edinburgh: Edinburgh University Press, 1978.

Ussery, Huling E. *Chaucer's Physician: Medicine and Literature in Fourteenth-Century England.* Tulane Studies in English 19. New Orleans: Department of English, Tulane University, 1971.

Veale, Elspeth M. "Craftsmen and the Economy of London in the Fourteenth Century." In *Studies in London History Presented to Philip Edmund Jones*, edited by A. E. J. Hollaender and William Kellaway, 133–51. London: Hodder and Stoughton, 1969.

Voigts, Linda E. "Anglo-Saxon Plant Remedies and the Anglo-Saxons." *Isis* 70 (1979): 250–68.

———. "Medical Prose." In *Middle English Prose: A Critical Guide to Major Authors and Genres*, edited by A. S. G. Edwards, 315–35. New Brunswick, N.J.: Rutgers University Press, 1984.

———. "Multitudes of Middle English Medical Manuscripts, or the Englishing of Science and Medicine." In *Manuscript Sources of Medieval Medicine: A Book of Essays*, edited by Margaret R. Schleissner, 183–95. New York: Garland Publishing, 1995.

———. "Scientific and Medical Books." In *Book Production and Publishing in Britain, 1375–1475*, edited by Jeremy Griffiths and Derek Pearsall, 345–402. Cambridge: Cambridge University Press, 1989.

Voigts, Linda E., and Robert P. Hudson. " 'A drynke that men callen dwale to make a man to slepe whyle men kerven him': A Surgical Anesthetic from Late Medieval England." In *Health, Disease and Healing in Medieval Culture*, edited by Sheila Campbell, Bert Hall, and David Klausner, 34–56. New York: St. Martin's Press, 1992.

Wack, Mary F. *Lovesickness in the Middle Ages: The* Viaticum *and Its Commentaries*. Philadelphia: University of Pennsylvania Press, 1990.

Walton, Michael T. "The Advisory Jury and Malpractice in 15th Century London: The Case of William Forest." *Journal of the History of Medicine* 40 (1985): 478–82.

Weiner, A. "A Note on Jewish Doctors in England in the Reign of Henry IV." *Jewish Quarterly Review* 18 (1905): 141–45.

Weisheipl, James A. "Curriculum of the Faculty of Arts at Oxford in the Early Fourteenth Century." *Mediaeval Studies* 26 (1964): 143–85.

———. "Science in the Thirteenth Century." In *The History of the University of Oxford*, vol. 1, *The Early Oxford Schools*, edited by J. I. Catto and T. A. R. Evans, 435–69. Oxford: Clarendon Press, 1984.

Weiss, Roberto. *Humanism in England during the Fifteenth Century*. 2d ed. Oxford: Basil Blackwell, 1957.

Welborn, Mary Catherine. "The Errors of the Doctors According to Friar Roger Bacon of the Minor Order." *Isis* 18 (1932): 26–62.

Wickersheimer, Ernest. *Dictionnaire biographique des médecins en France au moyen âge*. Paris: Librairie E. Droz, 1936.

Williams, Gwyn A. *Medieval London: From Commune to Capital*. London: Athlone Press, 1963.

Withington, E. "Roger Bacon and Medicine." In *Roger Bacon Essays*, edited by A. G. Little, 37–58. Oxford: Clarendon Press, 1914.

Ziegler, Philip. *The Black Death*. London: Collins, 1969.

Zier, Mark. "The Healing Power of the Hebrew Tongue: An Example from Late Thirteenth-Century England." In *Health, Disease and Healing in Medieval Culture*, edited by Sheila Campbell, Bert Hall, and David Klausner, 103–18. New York: St. Martin's Press, 1992.

Zimmermann, Volker. *Rezeption und Rolle der Heilkunde in landessprachigen handschriftlichen Kompendien des Spätmittelalters*. Stuttgart: Franz Steiner Verlag Wiesbaden, 1986.

Name Index

NOTE: Following the practice established in Talbot and Hammond, *The Medical Practitioners in Medieval England*, names of medieval persons are alphabetized by given name. All cross-references to "texts" refer to that entry in the Subject Index.

A. De Sutwell, Master, 119n.130
Adam, 55, 56
Adam (leper), 80
Adam Marsh, 26
Adam Rous, 50
Adam Tonworth, 66
Adams, J. N., 48
Adelard of Bath, 39
Albucasis, 119n.130. *See also* texts
Alexander Neckam, 39, 48. *See also* texts
Alexander of Tralles, 48, 115n.76, 119n.130. *See also* texts
Alfred, king of Anglo-Saxons, 47
Alfred of Sareshel, 16, 39, 42. *See also* texts
Alice Fizwaryn, 23
Alice le Pusere, 78
Alice Quernbetere, 73
Alice Ryvet, 74
Alice of Stocking, 7, 72
Alkyndi (al-Kindi), 59
Andrew le Sarazin, 77
Anthony Baldewyn, 29
Anthony de Romanis, 28
Aristotle, 17, 37, 38, 39, 40, 42, 43, 44, 48, 53, 54, 55, 57, 59, 68, 86. *See also* texts
Arnald of Villanova, 31, 119n.130. *See also* texts; texts—books
Arundel, earl of, 32
Augustine, Saint, 55
Averroes, 39, 50, 119n.130. *See also* texts
Avice, 11
Avicenna (Ibn Sina), 38, 39, 40, 43, 55, 57, 61, 67, 119n.130. *See also* texts

Bald (compiled Leechbook), 47
Baldwin, abbot of Bury, 24–25
Bardi, house of, 28
Bartholomew, Saint, 52
Bartholomew the Englishman (Bartholomaeus Anglicus), 16–17, 48–49, 52, 118n.127. *See also* texts

Bede (Venerable), 12–13, 20, 46. *See also* texts
Bernard Barbo, 30
Bernard Gordon, 18, 40, 44, 51, 119n.130. *See also* texts
Bertha Glanville, 80
Boccaccio, 87
Boethius, 89. *See also* texts
Bonaventura (chaplain), 99n.98
Bruno the Lombard, 119n.130. *See also* texts

Caelius Aurelianus, 46, 115n.76
Carlin, Martha, 90
Cassiodorus (senator), 46
Cassius Felix, 115n.76
Cato the Elder, 36, 45, 115n.79
Cecilia (*la leche*), 97n.55
Celsus, 45, 48
Charles the physician, 10
Christ, 7, 12, 41, 67, 89, 91
Christina Morel, 75
Cild (commissioned Leechbook), 116n.93
Clement VI, pope, 87
Cleupare (Cleopatra), 110n.15
Constantine the African, 17, 31, 38, 49, 119n.130. *See also* texts
Cook, Harold, 5
Cuthbert, Saint, 121–22n.168

David de Nigarellis de Lucca, 26
Deegan, Marilyn, 48
Demetrius de Cerno, 30
Dioscorides, 46, 55, 115n.76, 119n.130. *See also* texts

Eadricus (phlebotomist), 9
Edith Rogers of Wick, 78
Edward I, king of England, 22, 27, 29, 32, 52, 82, 104n.45
Edward II, king of England, husband of Isabella of France, 27, 28